LPN/LVN

State-Approved Schools *of* Nursing

1999

Meeting Minimum Requirements Set by Law and
Board Rules in the Various Jurisdictions

FORTY-FIRST EDITION

JONES AND BARTLETT PUBLISHERS
Sudbury, Massachusetts
BOSTON   TORONTO   LONDON   SINGAPORE

World Headquarters

Jones and Bartlett Publishers
40 Tall Pine Drive
Sudbury, MA 01776
978-443-5000
info@jbpub.com
www.jbpub.com

Jones and Bartlett Publishers International
Barb House, Barb Mews
London W6 7PA
UK

Jones and Bartlett Publishers Canada
2100 Bloor Street West
Suite 6-272
Toronto, ON M6S 5A5
CANADA

ISBN: 0-7637-1139-X

Printed in the United States of America
03 02 01 00   10 9 8 7 6 5 4 3 2 1

LPN/LVN
State-Approved
Schools *of* Nursing
1999

FORTY-FIRST EDITION

PREFACE

State-approved Schools of Nursing – LPN/LVN 1999 presents the NLN's Annual Survey of LPN/LVN Schools of Nursing, covering the period between October 16, 1997 and October 15, 1998. The publication provides a comprehensive listing of the more than 1,000 practical or vocational nursing programs in the U.S. and Puerto Rico, organized by State/Territory. The number of schools and programs in each State, the actual listing of programs, the list of new schools, and the list of those that closed during the specified time period are provided by the individual State Boards of Nursing and updated annually for inclusion in this publication.

Each school identified by the State Board is sent a survey to collect the following data for inclusion in this publication: address, telephone number, name and title of the director, NLNAC accreditation status, type of State Board approval, principal source of financial support for the program, and administrative control of the program. In addition, schools are asked to provide information about admissions, enrollments, graduations, program length, and admission requirements. A few schools have requested that specific information provided in the Annual Survey not be published, and such requests have been honored. Therefore, all the information presented here has been provided by the schools themselves and is made public with their permission.

Footnotes have been included in this publication to help the reader understand some of the new options available to the contemporary nursing student, as well as to clarify unusual features of some programs. You are encouraged to read the description of the footnotes that appears on page x.

A complete analysis of LPN/LVN data, including 10- to 20-year trends in statistics and data on men and minorities, will be published in the forthcoming ***Nursing DataSource, Volume III: Focus on Practical/Vocational Nursing***. Other volumes in the ***Nursing DataSource*** series that will be published in 2000 are ***Volume I: Trends in Contemporary RN Nursing Education*** and ***Volume II: Leaders in the Making: Graduate Education in Nursing***. In addition, the forthcoming compendium entitled ***Nursing Data Review*** presents findings from these Annual Surveys and other NLN research projects, including those related to recent graduates and nursing faculty.

We are confident that ***State-approved Schools of Nursing – LPN/LVN 1999*** will be a valuable resource to you. Please let us know what other sources of data about nursing programs, students, or faculty would be useful to you.

Theresa M. Valiga, Ed.D., R.N.
Director of Research and Professional Development
National League for Nursing

Contents

JURISDICTIONS INCLUDED
IN EACH GEOGRAPHIC REGION

Region 1
North Atlantic

16 Connecticut
51 Delaware
59 District of Columbia
11 Maine
14 Massachusetts
12 New Hampshire
22 New Jersey
21 New York
23 Pennsylvania
15 Rhode Island
13 Vermont

Region 2
Midwest

33 Illinois
32 Indiana
42 Iowa
47 Kansas
34 Michigan
41 Minnesota
43 Missouri
46 Nebraska
44 North Dakota
31 Ohio
45 South Dakota
35 Wisconsin

Region 3
Southern

63 Alabama
73 Arkansas
04 Canal Zone
58 Florida
57 Georgia
61 Kentucky
71 Louisiana
52 Maryland
64 Mississippi
55 North Carolina
74 Oklahoma
05 Puerto Rico
56 South Carolina
62 Tennessee
72 Texas
98 Virgin Island
53 Virginia
54 West Virginia

Region 4
Western

02 Alaska
94 American Samoa
85 Arizona
93 California
83 Colorado
89 Guam
01 Hawaii
88 Idaho
81 Montana
87 Nevada
84 New Mexico
92 Oregon
86 Utah
91 Washington
82 Wyoming

KEY TO ABBREVIATIONS AND SYMBOLS

Type of Program

HS - High School
HSE - High School Extended (includes high school plus some additional preparation)

NLNAC Accreditation as of January 31, 1999

A - Program accredited by the National League for Nursing Accrediting Commission

Administrative Control

SEC - Secondary school other than trade or technical
TCH - Trade, technical or vocational school or adult education center
COL - Senior college or university
CC - Junior or community college
HSP - Hospital
IND - Independent
GOV - Government agency other than hospital

Financial Support (principal source)

PBL - Public
PVT - Private

Publication Withheld - School has requested that publication of data be withheld

Educational Requirements for Entering Adult Program

10 - Tenth grade
11 - Eleventh grade
12 - Twelfth grade or GED

Other

ADN - Associate Degree in Nursing
AVTI - Adult Vocational- Technical Institute
BOCES - Board of Cooperative Educational Services
CETA - Comprehensive Employment and Training Act
CLG - Closing
HOE - Health Occupation Education
HOP(C) - Health Occupation Program (Center)
HSC - Health Science Center
JTPA - Job Training and Placement Program
L.P.N - Licensed Practical Nurse
L.V.N - Licensed Vocational Nurse
MDT(A) - Manpower Development and Training (Act)

FOOTNOTES

These footnotes are intended to identify special features of some programs. For more specific descriptions of these specific features, please contact the school directly.

Unless otherwise indicated with a footnote, all programs listed have full State Board approval.

1. Initial State Board approval

2. Provisional State Board approval

3. Experimental State Board approval

5. For Army personnel only. As of this year, all Army programs throughout the nation will report under US Army Academy of Health Science, Ft. Houston, TX.

6. Program is currently inactive ... Contact the school directly for more information

7. Program is affiliated with an Associate Degree program (See *State-Approved Schools of Nursing-RN)*

SCHOOLS OFFERING
L.P.N./L.V.N. PROGRAMS
IN THE VARIOUS JURISDICTIONS

School Code	Name of School, Director of Program, and Phone Number	Street Address City or Town and Zip Code		Footnotes	Type of Program	NLNAC Accreditation as of January 31, 1999	Administrative Control	Financial Support (principal source)	Number of Months in Program	Educational Requirements for Entering Adult Program	Enrollments as of October 15, 1998	Admissions Aug. 1, 1997 - July 31, 1998	Graduations Aug. 1, 1997 - July 31, 1998	Fall Admissions Aug. 1, 1998 - Dec. 31, 1998
	ALABAMA													
	23 Programs in 23 Schools													
023	AL Southern Comm College Mrs Margaret Denton, Chair *Chair's #: (334) 636-9642 Ext 658*	PO Box 489 Thomasville	36784				CC	PBL	16	12	50	91	44	32
026	Bessemer State Tech College Mrs Bobbie Daniel, Chair *Chair's #: (205) 428-6391 Ext 305*	PO Box 308 Bessemer	35020			A	TCH	PBL	16	12	138	137	84	52
025	Bevill State Comm College Mrs Alice Roberts, Asst Dean *Chair's #: (205) 648-3271 Ext 5430*	Drawer K PO Box 800 Sumiton	35148			A	CC	PBL			284	308	133	93
022	Bevill State Comm College Mrs Alice Roberts, Asst Dean *Chair's #: (205) 648-3271 Ext 5430*	Drawer 9 Highway 78 South Hamilton	35570			A	CC	PBL			Publication withheld			
007	Bishop State Comm College Ms Linda Shepherd, Dir *Chair's #: (334) 405-4495*	1365 Dr Martin L King Ave Mobile	36603				CC	PBL	16		127	91	91	54
019	Central AL Comm Coll Dr Melenie Bolton, Dir *Chair's #: (256) 249-5716*	PO Box 389 Childersburg	35044				CC	PBL			Publication withheld			
037	Chattahoochee Valley St Comm College Mrs Dixie Peterson, Chair *Chair's #: (334) 291-4925*	2602 College Dr Phenix City	36867	7			CC	PBL			Data reported w/AD prog			
020	Gadsden State Comm College Ms Tarva N Vaughn, Coord *Chair's #: (256) 549-8683*	PO Box 227 Gadsden	35901				CC	PBL			84	96	71	57
006	Harry M Ayers State Tech College Mrs Linda Cater, Chair *Chair's #: (256) 835-5400 Ext 517*	1801 Coleman Rd PO Box 164 Anniston	36201				TCH	PBL			Publication withheld			
015	J F Drake State Tech College Mrs Annice D Conaway, Dept Head *Chair's #: (256) 539-8161 Ext 129*	3421 Meridan St, N Huntsville	35811				TCH	PBL	14	12	79	119	46	51
008	John C Calhoun State Comm College Mrs Jane Floyd, Chair *Chair's #: (256) 306-2808*	PO Box 2216 Decatur	35602	7		A	CC	PBL			Data reported W/AD prog			
016	MacArthur State Tech College Mrs Sara M Goolsby, Chair *Chair's #: (334) 493-3573 Ext 275*	1708 N Main PO Box 910 Opp	36467				TCH	PBL	16	12	107	83	41	45
029	Northwest Shoal Comm Coll Mrs Suzie McCutcheon, Coord *Chair's #: (256) 331-5200*	PO Box 2545 Muscle Shoals	35660				TCH	PBL			Publication withheld			

Explanation of footnotes on page x

School Code	Name of School, Director of Program, and Phone Number	Street Address / City or Town and Zip Code	Footnotes	Type of Program	NLNAC Accreditation as of January 31, 1999	Administrative Control	Financial Support (principal source)	Number of Months in Program	Educational Requirements for Entering Adult Program	Enrollments as of October 15, 1998	Admissions Aug. 1, 1997 - July 31, 1998	Graduations Aug. 1, 1997 - July 31, 1998	Fall Admissions Aug. 1, 1998 - Dec. 31, 1998
	ALABAMA												
	- Continued												
024	Reid State Tech College Ms Patricia Gwin, Chair Chair's #: (334) 578-1313 Ext 124	PO Box 588 Evergreen 36401				TCH	PBL	16	12	105	88	94	21
009	Shelton State College Mrs Gladys Hill, Dir Chair's #: (205) 391-2445 Ext 2457	9500 Old Greensboro Rd Tuscaloosa 35405	7			TCH	PBL			Data reported w/AD prog			
034	Southern Comm College Mrs Beatrice Scruggs, Acting Dir Chair's #: (334) 727-5220	PO Box 830688 Tuskegee 36083			A	TCH	PVT			Publication withheld			
011	Southern Union State Comm College Mrs Regina Beaird, Chair Chair's #: (334) 756-4151 Ext 5249	321 Fob James Drive Valley 36854			A	CC	PBL	12	12	63	49	31	35
027	Sparks State Tech College Mrs Sherry Barnes, Dir Chair's #: (334) 687-3543 Ext 273	PO Drawer 580 Eufaula 36072				TCH	PBL			Publication withheld			
028	Trenholm State Tech College PN Prog Mrs Annitta Love, Director Chair's #: (334) 240-9655	1225 Air Base Blvd Montgomery 36108			A	TCH	PBL	15	12	113	246	77	54
005	Wallace Community College Dr Belinda Wendy Downing, Dir Chair's #: (334) 983-3521 Ext 263	Route 6 Box 62 Dothan 36303			A	CC	PBL	12	12	144	163	64	67
030	Wallace St Comm College Mrs Denise Elliott, Dir Chair's #: (256) 352-8198	PO Box 2000 Hanceville 35077	7			CC	PBL	12	12	50	72	45	63
018	Wallace St Comm College Dr Sheila Guidry, Dir Chair's #: (334) 876-9338	PO Drawer 1049 Selma 36701			A	CC	PBL	15	12	64	98	44	64
	AMERICAN SAMOA												
	1 Program in 1 School												
001	American Samoa Comm College-PN Pro Mrs Lele Ah-Mu Magep, Chair Chair's #: (684) 699-9156	Mapusaga Pago Pago 96799				CC	PBL			Publication withheld			
	ARIZONA												
	19 Programs in 13 Schools												
019	Arizona Western College Ms Judy Jondahl, Director Chair's #: (520) 344-7798	PO Box 929 Yuma 85364	7			CC	PBL	11	12	40	40	16	40
008	Central AZ College-Signal Peak Campus Dr Eleanor Strang, Director Chair's #: (520) 426-4330 Ext 4331	8470 N Overfield Rd Coolidge 85228	7			CC	PBL			Data reported w/AD prog			

Explanation of footnotes on page x

School Code	Name of School, Director of Program, and Phone Number	Street Address City or Town and Zip Code	Footnotes	Type of Program	NLNAC Accreditation as of January 31, 1999	Administrative Control	Financial Support (principal source)	Number of Months in Program	Educational Requirements for Entering Adult Program	Enrollments as of October 15, 1998	Admissions Aug. 1, 1997 - July 31, 1998	Graduations Aug. 1, 1997 - July 31, 1998	Fall Admissions Aug. 1, 1998 - Dec. 31, 1998
	ARIZONA												
	- Continued												
005	Cochise College Ms Susan Macdonald, Interim Dir Chair's #: (520) 364-0310	4190 West Highway 80 Douglas 85607	7			CC	PBL			Data reported w/AD Prog			
011	Gateway Comm College (2 Branches) Mrs Frieda Muwakkil, Dir Chair's #: (602) 392-5088	PO Box 13349 Phoenix 85004				CC	PBL	8	12	105	59	67	57
018	Maricopa Skill Ctr Ms Sue Elenbaas, Coord Chair's #: (602) 238-4369	1245 E Buckeye Rd Phoenix 85034				TCH	PBL			Publication withheld			
007	Mesa Comm College (2 Branches) Ms Myrba Eshelman, Chair Chair's #: (602) 461-7108	1833 W Southern Ave Mesa 85202	7			CC	PBL			Data reported w/AD prog			
001	Metro Tech/Voc Inst of Phoenix Mrs Shar n A Pearce, Director Chai s #: (602) 271-2650	1900 W Thomas Rd Phoenix 85015		HS		SEC SEC	PBL PBL	9		11 17	10 27	6 10	13 27
009	Mohave Comm College Dr Sharon Hays, Dir Chair's #: (520) 757-0863	1971 Jagerson Ave Kingman 86401	7			CC	PBL			Data reported w/AD prog			
016	Phoenix College Dr Daniel Tetting, Chair Chair's #: (602) 285-7128	1202 West Thomas Rd Phoenix 85013	7			CC	PBL			Data reported w/AD prog			
013	Pima Comm College Ms Vonnie Erickson, Dir Chair's #: (520) 206-6661	2202 W Anklam Rd Tucson 85709				CC	PBL			Publication withheld			
010	Pima Comm College Mrs Emelia Lewis, Coord Chair's #: (520) 206-5113	5901 So Calle Santa Cruz Tucson 85709				CC	PBL	13	12	18	48	41	35
002	Scottsdale Comm Coll Ms Nellie Nelson, Chair Chair's #: (602) 423-6226	9000 E Chapparral Rd Scottsdale 85256	7			CC	PBL			Data reported w/AD Prog			
015	Yavapai College Dr Lynn Nugent, Div Chair Chair's #: (602) 445-7300	1100 East Sheldon St Prescott 86301	7			CC	PBL			Data reported w/AD prog			
	ARKANSAS												
	29 Programs in 29 Schools												
017	Arkansas Valley Tech Inst Ms Elizabeth Pruitt, Chair Chair's #: (501) 667-2117	PO Box 17000 Fort Smith 72917				TCH	PBL	11	12	62	80	60	40

School Code	Name of School, Director of Program, and Phone Number	Street Address / City or Town and Zip Code	Footnotes	Type of Program	NLNAC Accreditation as of January 31, 1999	Administrative Control	Financial Support (principal source)	Number of Months in Program	Educational Requirements for Entering Adult Program	Enrollments as of October 15, 1998	Admissions Aug. 1, 1997 - July 31, 1998	Graduations Aug. 1, 1997 - July 31, 1998	Fall Admissions Aug. 1, 1998 - Dec. 31, 1998
	ARKANSAS												
	- Continued												
052	ASU Mt Home Miss Victoria Oxner, Chair *Chair's #: (870) 425-3949 Ext 234*	213 E 6th St Mt Home 72653				COL	PBL	11	12	19	44	12	24
031	ASU-Newport Mrs Paula Breckenridge, Chair *Chair's #: (870) 523-8966 Ext 0020*	PO Box 1120 Newport 72112				CC	PBL	Publication withheld					
002	Baptist Sch of PN Dr Shirlene Harris, Dir *Chair's #: (501) 202-7402 Ext 7433*	11900 Colonel Glenn Rd Little Rock 72210			A	HSP	PVT	12	12	35	77	52	77
030	Black River Tech Coll Ms Loretta Dismang, Chair *Chair's #: (870) 892-4565 Ext 256*	PO Box 468 Pocahontas 72455				CC	PBL	Publication withheld					
032	Cossatot Tech Coll Mrs Kay Lockhard, Instructor *Chair's #: (860) 584-4471 Ext 26*	PO Box 960 De Queen 71832				TCH	PBL			40	40	37	40
029	Cotton Boll Tech Inst Ms Kathy Evans, Chair *Chair's #: (870) 239-3200*	4601 Lindwood Dr Burdette 72321				TCH	PBL	11	12	20	20	14	20
014	Crowley's Ridge Tech Inst Mrs Mary Wallace, Chair *Chair's #: (870) 391-3369 Ext 19*	PO Box 925 Forrest City 72335				TCH	PBL	Publication withheld					
004	Delta Tech Inst Mrs Kathleen Brewer, Chair *Chair's #: (870) 932-2176 Ext 13*	2916 Willow Rd Jonesboro 72401				TCH	PBL	11	12	40	44	41	27
022	Foothills Tech Inst Ms Gail Burton, Chair *Chair's #: (501) 207-4035*	1800 E Moore Ave Searcy 72143				TCH	PBL	11	12	24	30	16	26
041	Forest Echoes Tech Inst Ms Sheila Upshaw, Chair *Chair's #: (870) 364-6414*	1326 Highway 52 W Crossett 71635				TCH	PBL	Publication withheld					
035	Great Rivers Vo Tech School Ms D Boyter Evans, Chair *Chair's #: (870) 222-5360 Ext 222*	PO Box 747 1609 E Ash St McGehee 71654				TCH	PBL	Publication withheld					
042	Mid-South Comm College Mrs Gale Allen, Chair *Chair's #: (501) 733-6773*	PO Box 2067 West Memphis 72301				CC	PBL	Publication withheld					
013	North Arkansas College Mrs Mary Wallace, Chair *Chair's #: (870) 391-3369*	Pioneer Ridge Harrison 72602			A	TCH	PBL	11	12	24	42	22	17

Explanation of footnotes on page x

School Code	Name of School, Director of Program, and Phone Number	Street Address, City or Town and Zip Code	Footnotes	Type of Program	NLNAC Accreditation as of January 31, 1999	Administrative Control	Financial Support (principal source)	Number of Months in Program	Educational Requirements for Entering Adult Program	Enrollments as of October 15, 1998	Admissions Aug. 1, 1997 - July 31, 1998	Graduations Aug. 1, 1997 - July 31, 1998	Fall Admissions Aug. 1, 1998 - Dec. 31, 1998
	ARKANSAS												
	- Continued												
009	Northwest Tech Inst Mrs Ruth Jones, Chair Chair's #: (501) 751-8824 Ext 112	709 S Old Missouri Rd Springdale 72765				TCH	PBL			45	51	36	48
037	Ouachita Tech College Ms Lynette Smith, Chair Chair's #: (501) 332-3658 Ext 52	PO Box 816 Malvern 72104				TCH	PBL	12	12	24	20	15	25
028	Ozarka Tech College Ms Kitty Smith, Chair Chair's #: (870) 368-7371 Ext 325	PO Box 10 Melbourne 72556				TCH	PBL	18	12	32	16	16	18
016	Petit Jean Coll Ms Carol Loyd, Chair Chair's #: (501) 354-2465	#1 Bruce Morrilton 72110				TCH	PBL			Publication withheld			
033	Phillips Comm Coll Ms Hazel Smith, Coord Chair's #: (870) 946-3506 Ext 1611	PO Box 427 Dewitt 72042				CC	PBL			Publication withheld			
001	Pulaski Tech Coll Ms Sherry Bowman, Dir Chair's #: (501) 812-2235	3000 W Scenic Rd N Little Rock 72118				CC	PBL	11	12	30	30	23	30
008	Quapaw Tech Inst Ms Betty Haygood, Chair Chair's #: (501) 767-9314 Ext 352	PO Box 3950 200 Mid America Hot Springs 71914				TCH	PBL	11	12	34	47	21	44
034	Rich Mountain Comm College PN Prog Mrs Charla Hollin, Dir Chair's #: (501) 394-7622 Ext 1366	1100 Bush St Mena 71953				CC	PBL			Publication withheld			
051	SAU Tech Mrs Janet Grace, Chair Chair's #: (870) 574-4498	100 Carr Rd E Camden 71701				CC	PBL	10	12	27	27	14	29
019	South AR Comm College Miss Betty F Owen, Chair Chair's #: (870) 864-7118 Ext 234	PO Box 7010 El Dorado 71731				CC	PBL	12	12	44	50	46	25
006	Southeast AR College Mrs Diann W Williams, Coord Chair's #: (870) 543-5929	1900 Hazel St Pine Bluff 71603				TCH	PBL			Publication withheld			
020	Univ of AR Comm Coll Mrs Laura Massey, Chair Chair's #: (870) 777-5722 Ext 278	PO Box 140 Hwy 295 Hope 71801				CC	PBL			24	0	21	26
011	Univ of AR Comm Coll Ms Dawn Stueve, Chair Chair's #: (870) 793-7581 Ext 0025	PO Box 3350 Batesville 72501				CC	PBL	11	12	27	24	16	20

Explanation of footnotes on page x

School Code	Name of School, Director of Program, and Phone Number	Street Address — City or Town and Zip Code	Footnotes	Type of Program	NLNAC Accreditation as of January 31, 1999	Administrative Control	Financial Support (principal source)	Number of Months in Program	Educational Requirements for Entering Adult Program	Enrollments as of October 15, 1998	Admissions Aug. 1, 1997 - July 31, 1998	Graduations Aug. 1, 1997 - July 31, 1998	Fall Admissions Aug. 1, 1998 - Dec. 31, 1998
	ARKANSAS												
	- Continued												
010	Westark College PN Prog Ms Kathy J Redding, Dir *Chair's #: (501) 788-7376*	Box 3649 Fort Smith 72913				CC	PBL	12	12	14	59	20	14
	CALIFORNIA												
	89 Programs in 76 Schools												
089	Allan Hancock College Ms deBechevet, Interim AssocDean *Chair's #: (805) 922-6966 Ext 3383*	800 S College Dr Santa Maria 93454	7			CC	PBL			Data Reported w/AD prog			
023	American Career College Mrs Diane Neville, Dir *Chair's #: (323) 906-2207 Ext 207*	4021 Rosewood Ave Los Angeles 90004				TCH	PVT			Publication withheld			
047	Antelope Valley College Ms Sue Albert, Interim Dean *Chair's #: (661) 722-6402*	3041 W Avenue K Lancaster 93536				CC	PBL			29	0	11	30
004	Bakersfield College-Dept of Nsg, Ms Sheran DeLeon, Dir *Chair's #: (805) 395-4281*	1801 Panorama Dr Bakersfield 93305				CC	PBL			34	45	17	0
087	Butte Jr College Dist Ms Lynn Phillips, Director *Chair's #: (530) 895-2328*	3536 Butte Campus Dr Oroville 95965				CC	PBL			Publication withheld			
053	Cabrillo College-VN Dept Mrs Joan Frommhagern, Dir *Chair's #: (831) 479-6280*	6500 Soquel Dr Aptos 95003				CC	PBL			Publication withheld			
716	Casa Loma College (2 Campuses) Ms Maryann Frauenholz, Director *Chair's #: (213) 290-6440*	6850 Van Nuys Blvd Suite 318 Van Nuys 91405			A	TCH	PVT			Publication withheld			
728	Cerro Coso Comm College Ms Mary T Kowalski, Dir *Chair's #: (760) 384-6333*	3000 College Heights Blvd Ridgecrest 93555				CC	PBL	18	12	14	15	14	15
024	Chaffey College Mrs S Dawson, Dir *Chair's #: (909) 941-2695 Ext 2695*	5885 Haven Ave Rancho Cucamonga 91737				CC	PBL	18	12	36	45	22	41
081	Citrus College Mrs Marilyn Collins, Dept Chair *Chair's #: (626) 914-8721*	1000 W Foothill Blvd Glendora 91741				CC	PBL			Publication withheld			
020	City College of San Francisco Mrs Evelyn Massey Porter, Dir *Chair's #: (415) 561-1912*	1860 Hayes St San Francisco 94117				CC	PBL			Publication withheld			

Explanation of footnotes on page x

Explanation of footnotes on page x

CALIFORNIA

- Continued

School Code	Name of School, Director of Program, and Phone Number	Street Address, City or Town and Zip Code	Footnotes	Type of Program	NLNAC Accreditation as of January 31, 1999	Administrative Control	Financial Support (principal source)	Number of Months in Program	Educational Requirements for Entering Adult Program	Enrollments as of October 15, 1998	Admissions Aug. 1, 1997 - July 31, 1998	Graduations Aug. 1, 1997 - July 31, 1998	Fall Admissions Aug. 1, 1998 - Dec. 31, 1998
745	Clovis Adult Sch & Voc Ed — Mrs Lola L Gasperetti, Director — Chair's #: (559) 298-2172	1452 David E Cook Way — Clovis 92611				SEC	PBL			Publication withheld			
712	Coll of the Canyons — Dr Kathleen Welch, Dir — Chair's #: (805) 259-7800 Ext 3366	26455 N Rockwell Canyon — Valencia 91355	7			CC	PBL			Data reported w/AD prog			
075	Coll of the Desert (2 Campuses) — Mrs Celia Hartley, Chair — Chair's #: (760) 773-2580	43-500 Monterey Ave — Palm Desert 92260				CC	PBL	12	12	30	49	41	39
045	Coll of the Redwoods (3 Campuses) — Ms S Stuart-Siddall, Dir — Chair's #: (707) 476-4216	7351 Thompkins Hill Rd — Eureka 95501				CC	PBL	12	12	25	30	55	25
708	Coll of the Siskiyous — Mrs Gerri L Fedora, Director — Chair's #: (530) 938-5270	800 College Ave — Weed 96094				CC	PBL			Publication withheld			
029	Compton College — Dr Roberta West, Dean — Chair's #: (310) 900-1600 Ext 2700	1111 E Artesia Blvd — Compton 90221	7			CC	PBL			Data reported w/AD prog			
044	Compton Unified Sch Dist — Ms Lillian Giles, Dir — Chair's #: (310) 603-1829	3663 Martin Luther King Blvd — Lynwood 90262				GOV	PBL			Publication withheld			
098	Concorde Career Inst — Ms Jean Stephemor, Dir — Chair's #: (909) 884-8891 Ext 24	570 W 4th St — San Bernardino 92401				TCH	PVT			Publication withheld			
010	Concorde Career Inst — Mrs Muriel Owen, Dir — Chair's #: (619) 688-0800 Ext 0032	123 Camino De La Reina — San Diego 92108				TCH	PVT	12	12	22	30	25	11
085	Concorde Career Inst-Valley College — Mrs Georgene Tacke, Dir — Chair's #: (818) 766-8151 Ext 252	12412 Victory Blvd — North Hollywood 95823				TCH	PVT			180	210	190	60
005	Concorde Career Institute — Chriss Benvenuti, Director — Chair's #: (714) 635-3450	1717 South Brookhurst — Anaheim 92840				TCH	PVT			Publication withheld			
055	De Anza Comm Coll — Mrs Georgeanne Adamy, Dept Head — Chair's #: (408) 864-8775	21250 Stevens Creek Blvd — Cupertino 95014	7			CC	PBL			Data reported w/AD prog			
035	Emanuel Turlock PN Prog — Mrs Judith Black, Director — Chair's #: (209) 669-2305	825 Delbon Ave — Turlock 95380				TCH	PBL			Publication withheld			

School Code	Name of School, Director of Program, and Phone Number	Street Address / City or Town and Zip Code	Footnotes	Type of Program	NLNAC Accreditation as of January 31, 1999	Administrative Control	Financial Support (principal source)	Number of Months in Program	Educational Requirements for Entering Adult Program	Enrollments as of October 15, 1998	Admissions Aug. 1, 1997 - July 31, 1998	Graduations Aug. 1, 1997 - July 31, 1998	Fall Admissions Aug. 1, 1998 - Dec. 31, 1998
	CALIFORNIA												
	- Continued												
067	Four D Success Academy Dr Cherry Houston, Dir *Chair's #: (800) 600-5422*	952 So Mt Vernon Suite B Calton 92324				TCH	PBL			Publication withheld			
094	Gavilan College Mrs Kay Bedell, Director *Chair's #: (408) 848-4883*	5055 Santa Teresa Blvd Gilroy 95020				CC	PBL	24	12	29	24	12	8
011	Glendale Career College Ms Jean Nix, Dir *Chair's #: (818) 243-1131 Ext 263*	1015 Grandview Ave Glendale 91201				TCH	PVT	14	12	113	180	145	45
030	Glendale College Dr Sharon Hall, Assoc Dean *Chair's #: (818) 551-5270*	1500 N Verdugo Rd Glendale 91208				CC	PBL	12	12	33	44	27	23
749	Grant Adult & Comm Ed Mrs Maxine Times, Director *Chair's #: (916) 263-6511*	3701 Stephen Dr N Highlands 95660				TCH	PBL			Publication withheld			
046	Grossmont Hlth Occupations Center Mrs B Patricia Twyman, Director *Chair's #: (619) 596-3665*	9368 Oakbourne Rd Santee 92071				SEC	PBL	15	12	65	0	45	68
741	Hacienda-La Puente Adult Educ Mrs Elda Pichetto, Dir *Chair's #: (616) 855-3138*	15325 E Los Robles Hacienda Heights 91745				TCH	PBL	12	12	53	59	49	30
077	Hanford Adult School (2 Campuses) Mrs Karen Ormsby, Director *Chair's #: (559) 583-0856 Ext 3524*	120 E Grangeville Blvd Hanford 93230				SEC	PBL	13	12	40	32	52	21
039	Hartnell College Mrs Chirs Eatom, Director *Chair's #: (408) 755-6771*	156 Homestead Ave Salinas 93901				CC	PBL			Publication withheld			
060	Imperial Valley College Dr Betty Marks, Admin *Chair's #: (760) 352-8320*	PO Box 158 Imperial 92251				CC	PBL			Publication withheld			
736	Lassen Comm College Ms Liona Maas, Dir *Chair's #: (530) 251-8820*	PO Box 3000 Susanville 96130				CC	PBL			Publication withheld			
071	Long Beach City College Mrs Verla Beck, Dir *Chair's #: (562) 938-4101*	4901 E Carson St Long Beach 90808				CC	PBL	12	12	125	90	90	45
013	Los Angeles Trade-Tech Coll-VN Prog Mrs Pat Merrill, Director *Chair's #: (213) 744-9452*	400 W Washington Blvd Los Angeles 90015				CC	PBL	15	12	87	30	33	25

Explanation of footnotes on page x

School Code	Name of School, Director of Program, and Phone Number	Street Address City or Town and Zip Code	Footnotes	Type of Program	NLNAC Accreditation as of January 31, 1999	Administrative Control	Financial Support (principal source)	Number of Months in Program	Educational Requirements for Entering Adult Program	Enrollments as of October 15, 1998	Admissions Aug. 1, 1997 - July 31, 1998	Graduations Aug. 1, 1997 - July 31, 1998	Fall Admissions Aug. 1, 1998 - Dec. 31, 1998
	CALIFORNIA												
	- Continued												
719	Los Angeles Unified Sch District Mrs Lillian Goodman, Director Chair's #: (213) 625-6649	1320 W 3rd St, Rm 216 Los Angeles 90017				TCH	PBL			90	105	95	90
027	Los Medanos College Ms Elizabeth Coats, Dir Chair's #: (925) 439-2181	2700 E Leland Rd Pittsburg 94565				CC	PBL			27	30	25	30
748	Lynwood Adult Sch Mrs Elizabeth McCray, Dir Chair's #: (310) 604-1786	12124 Bullis Rd Lynwood 90262				SEC	PBL			Publication withheld			
072	Marian College Mrs Cirlezita Cabote, Dir Chair's #: (213) 388-3566	3325 Wishire Blvd Suite 1213 Los Angeles 90010				TCH	PVT	12	12	23	16	16	23
739	Maric College (2 Campuses) Mrs Phyllis Crownover, Dir Chair's #: (619) 279-4500	3666 Kearny Villa Rd San Diego 92123				TCH	PVT			Publication withheld			
043	Merced College Ms Penny Sawyer, Dir Chair's #: (209) 384-6128	3600 M St Merced 95348				CC	PBL	18	12	32	36	26	0
003	Merritt College Mrs Carol A Lee, Director Chair's #: (510) 436-2506	12500 Campus Dr Oakland 94619	7			CC	PBL			Data reported w/AD prog			
733	Metropolitan Ed Dist Ms Meg Stanley, Director Chair's #: (408) 723-6400 Ext 509	760 Hillsdale Ave San Jose 95136				TCH	PBL	12	12	26	29	30	0
073	Mira Costa College Ms Katherine M Herd, Director Chair's #: (760) 795-6842	One Barnard Dr Oceanside 92056				CC	PBL	18	12	38	80	23	15
083	Mission College Ms Ann Cowels, Chair Chair's #: (408) 748-2748	3000 Mission College Blvd Santa Clara 95054				CC	PBL			90	60	56	30
062	Mt San Jacinto College Mrs Judy Gentry, Dir Chair's #: (909) 672-6752 Ext 2609	28237 La Piedra Rd Menifee 92584				CC	PBL			Publication withheld			
015	Napa Valley College Ms Patty Vail, Dean Chair's #: (707) 253-3120	2277 Napa-Vallejo Hwy Napa 94558				CC	PBL	12	12	68	45	35	0
012	NCP Voc School Mrs Nelly Jacson, Director Chair's #: (650) 871-0701	881 Sneath Lane San Bruno 94066	1			TCH	PBL			Publication withheld			

Explanation of footnotes on page x

School Code	Name of School, Director of Program, and Phone Number	Street Address, City or Town and Zip Code	Footnotes	Type of Program	NLNAC Accreditation as of January 31, 1999	Administrative Control	Financial Support (principal source)	Number of Months in Program	Educational Requirements for Entering Adult Program	Enrollments as of October 15, 1998	Admissions Aug. 1, 1997 - July 31, 1998	Graduations Aug. 1, 1997 - July 31, 1998	Fall Admissions Aug. 1, 1998 - Dec. 31, 1998
	CALIFORNIA												
	- Continued												
746	North Orange County ROP Mrs Janine O' Buchon, Director *Chair's #: (714)502-5950 Ext 14*	1617 E Ball Rd Anaheim 92805				TCH	PBL	12	12	89	120	84	60
099	Oxnard Adult Sch-Voc Prog Dr Dorothy Phillips, Coord *Chair's #: (805) 388-8145*	280 Skyway Dr Commarita 93010				SEC	PBL			Publication withheld			
074	Pacific College Mrs Judy Beem, Director *Chair's #: (714) 662-4402*	3160 Redhill Ave Costa Mesa 92626	1			CC	PBL			Publication withheld			
058	Palo Verde Comm Coll Ms Diane Dumas, Assoc Dean *Chair's #: (760) 921-5344*	811 West Chanslorway Blythe 92225				CC	PBL	18	12	19	15	0	0
001	Pasadena City College Ms Mary Wynn, Dean *Chair's #: (626) 585-7323*	1570 E Colorado Blvd Pasadena 91106	7			CC	PBL			Data reported w/AD prog			
705	Pittsburg Adult Ed Mrs Bridget P Teranen, Director *Chair's #: (925) 473-4460*	1151 Stoneman Ave Pittsburg 94565				TCH	PBL			Publication withheld			
750	Plumas & Sierra Counties ROP Mr Paul Mrowcznski, Director *Chair's #: (916) 283-6500 Ext 213*	50 Church St Suite B Quincy 95971				TCH	PBL			Publication withheld			
082	Porterville College Ms Valerie Lombardi, Dir *Chair's #: (559) 791-2322*	100 E College Ave Porterville 93257				CC	PBL			45	30	26	15
751	Poway Unified Sch Dist ROP Mrs Nancy A Allen, Director *Chair's #: (619) 679-0158*	12450 Glenoak Rd Poway 92064				SEC	PBL			23	23	0	0
735	Redlands Unified Sch Dist-Adult Sch Ms Pam Hinckley, Chair *Chair's #: (909) 307-5315*	7 West Delaware Ave Redlands 92373				TCH	PBL	17	12	53	60	20	0
063	Rio Hondo Jr College Mrs Marcia McCormick, Dir *Chair's #: (562) 692-0921 Ext 3596*	3600 Workman Mill Rd Whittier 90601	7			CC	PBL			Data reported w/AD prog			
017	Riverside Comm College Dr D Abrashoff Schutte, Dir *Chair's #: (909) 222-8408*	4800 Magnolia Ave Riverside 92506				CC	PBL	12	12	86	68	50	59
033	Sacramento City College VN Prog Mrs Diane Welch, Dir *Chair's #: (916) 558-2275*	3835 Freeport Blvd Sacramento 95822				CC	PBL	18	12	20	40	30	20

Explanation of footnotes on page x

CALIFORNIA

- Continued

School Code	Name of School, Director of Program, and Phone Number	Street Address / City or Town and Zip Code	Footnotes	Type of Program	NLNAC Accreditation as of January 31, 1999	Administrative Control	Financial Support (principal source)	Number of Months in Program	Educational Requirements for Entering Adult Program	Enrollments as of October 15, 1998	Admissions Aug. 1, 1997 - July 31, 1998	Graduations Aug. 1, 1997 - July 31, 1998	Fall Admissions Aug. 1, 1998 - Dec. 31, 1998
066	San Bernardino Adult School / Ms Pam Hinckley, Dir / Chair's #: (909) 388-6052	1200 N "E" St / San Bernardino 92405				TCH	PBL			Publication withheld			
036	San Joaquin Delta Comm College / Ms Debra Lewis, Dir / Chair's #: (209) 954-5516	5151 Pacific Ave / Stockton 95207				CC	PBL	12	12	29	30	30	0
084	San Joaquin Valley College / Ms Beberly Breedveld, Dir / Chair's #: (559(651-2500 Ext 152	8400 W Mineral King Ave / Visalia 73291	1			CC	PVT			Publication withheld			
048	Santa Barbara City College / Ms Jacqueline Huth, Director / Chair's #: (805) 965-0581 Ext 2233	721 Cliff Dr / Santa Barbara 93109				CC	PBL	18	12	19	28	18	0
042	Santa Rosa Jr College / Ms Joan Scarborough, Director / Chair's #: (707) 527-4529	1501 Mendocino Dr / Santa Rosa 95401				CC	PBL	18	12	29	31	23	0
026	Shasta College / Ms Georgianne Dinkel, Director / Chair's #: (530) 225-4725	11555 Old OR Trail / Redding 96049				CC	PBL			29	30	30	0
054	Sierra College / Ms Margaret White, Assoc Dean / Chair's #: (916) 781-0556	5000 Rocklin Rd / Rocklin 95677				CC	PBL			Publication withheld			
092	Simi Vly Adult Sch / Mrs Lois Harrion, Dir / Chair's #: (805) 579-6260	3192 Los Angeles Ave / Simi Valley 93065				TCH	PBL			17	23	21	18
069	Southwestern College / Ms Charlotte A Erdahl, Dean	900 Otay Lakes Rd / Chula Vista 91910				CC	PBL	18	12	22	42	0	0
097	St Francis Career Coll / Mrs Marilyn Overby, Dir / Chair's #: (310) 603-1830	3630 E Imperial Highway / Lynwood 90262				TCH	PVT			28	66	48	26
037	Summit Career College / Dr Sybil Damon, Director / Chair's #: (909) 422-8950	1330 E Cooley Dr / Colton 92324				TCH	PVT			Publication withheld			
019	Tri -Co ROP Voc Nursing Prog / Mrs Pamela Mahmoudi, Dir / Chair's #: (530) 822-3236	256 Wilbur Ave / Yuba 95992	1			TCH	PBL	19	12	28	29	0	0
079	Ukiah Adult Sch Voc Nsg Prog / Mrs Ruby Rose, Director / Chair's #: (707) 463-5217	1056 N Bush St / Ukiah 95482				TCH	PBL	14	12	27	36	0	0

Explanation of footnotes on page x

School Code	Name of School, Director of Program, and Phone Number	Street Address City or Town and Zip Code		Footnotes	Type of Program	NLNAC Accreditation as of January 31, 1999	Administrative Control	Financial Support (principal source)	Number of Months in Program	Educational Requirements for Entering Adult Program	Enrollments as of October 15, 1998	Admissions Aug. 1, 1997 - July 31, 1998	Graduations Aug. 1, 1997 - July 31, 1998	Fall Admissions Aug. 1, 1998 - Dec. 31, 1998
	CALIFORNIA													
	- Continued													
080	Visalia Adult Sch Mr Dennis Lukehart, Director Chair's #: (209) 730-7655	3110 Houston Ave Visalia	93277	1			TCH	PBL	13	12	28	34	29	30
056	Western Career College Ms Debra Aucoin-Ratcliff, Dir Chair's #: (916) 361-1660 Ext 714	8909 Folson Blvd Sacramento	95826				TCH	PVT	18	12	61	73	32	0
040	Yuba College Ms Margot Loschke, Director Chair's #: (916) 741-6785	2088 N Beale Rd Marysville	95901				CC	PBL			30	25	16	0
078	YWCA Los Angeles Job Corps Ctr Miss Evangeline Malabanan, Dir Chair's #: (213) 741-5316	1106 S Broadway Los Angeles	90015				GOV	PBL			Publication withheld			
	COLORADO													
	17 Programs in 17 Schools													
006	Colorado Mountain College Dr N Kuhrik, Director Chair's #: (970) 945-7486 Ext 6240	3000 County Rd 114 Glenwood Spring	81601	1			CC	PBL			Publication withheld			
026	Comm College of Denver Mrs Vicki V Earnest, Coord Chair's #: (303) 556-3842	PO Box 173363 Denver	80217	7			CC	PBL			Data reported w/AD prog			
005	Concorde Career Institute Ms Jacqueline Verville, Dir Chair's #: (303) 832-1690	770 Grant St Denver	80203				TCH	PVT	13	12	88	93	68	45
021	Delta Montrose Area Voc Tech Sch Mrs Shari Barclay, Coord Chair's #: (970) 874-7671 Ext 121	1765 US Hwy 50 Delta	81416				TCH	PBL	9	12	35	26	20	26
002	Emily Griffith Opportunity School Dr E Ford-Pade, Dir Chair's #: (303) 575-4737	1250 Welton St Lakewood	80226				TCH	PBL			Publication withheld			
017	FRCC/Larimer County Center Ms Rebecca Lynch, Coord Chair's #: (970) 204-8223 Ext 203	4616 S Shields Fort Collins	80526	7			CC	PBL			Data reported w/AD prog			
013	Front Range Comm Coll Mrs Medrrilee McDffie, Director Chair's #: (303) 516-8917	2255 N Main St Longmont	80501				CC	PBL	9	12	39	37	30	32
029	Front Range Comm College Mrs Alma L Mueller, Dir Chair's #: (303) 404-5202	3645 W 112th Ave Westminster	80030	7			CC	PBL			Data reported w/AD prog			

Explanation of footnotes on page x

School Code	Name of School, Director of Program, and Phone Number	Street Address	City or Town and Zip Code	Footnotes	Type of Program	NLNAC Accreditation as of January 31, 1999	Administrative Control	Financial Support (principal source)	Number of Months in Program	Educational Requirements for Entering Adult Program	Enrollments as of October 15, 1998	Admissions Aug. 1, 1997 - July 31, 1998	Graduations Aug. 1, 1997 - July 31, 1998	Fall Admissions Aug. 1, 1998 - Dec. 31, 1998
	COLORADO													
	- Continued													
010	Lamar Comm College Ms Sandy Summers, Dir *Chair's #: (719) 336-2248 Ext 415*	2401 South Main St Lamar	81052				TCH	PBL			Publication withheld			
015	Northeastern Jr College, PN Prog Ms Betty Brunner, Coord *Chair's #: (970) 521-6749 Ext 6749*	100 College St Sterling	80751				CC	PBL	11	12	30	24	19	25
028	Otero Jr College Mrs Denise Root, Dir *Chair's #: (719) 384-6894*	La Junta	81050	7			CC	PBL			Data reported w/AD prog			
009	Pueblo Comm College (2 Branches) Mrs Jan Lewis, Chair *Chair's #: (719) 549-3284 Ext 3279*	900 W Orman Pueblo	81004			A	TCH	PBL			Publication withheld			
027	San Juan Basin Tech Sch Mrs Nancy Brown, Dir *Chair's #: (970) 385-4267 Ext 129*	Po Box 970 Cortez	81321				TCH	PBL			27	31	28	28
016	T H Pickens Ctr/Aurora Public Schs Ms Paula Barnaby, Dir *Chair's #: (303) 344-4910*	500 Buckley Rd Aurora	80011				TCH	PBL			Publication withheld			
008	Trinidad State Jr College Sch of PN Ms Judie E Stickel, Director *Chair's #: (719) 846-5524*	600 Prospect St Trinidad	81082				CC	PBL			Publication withheld			
	CONNECTICUT													
	12 Programs in 12 Schools													
053	A I Prince Voc Techs Sch Mrs Gayle Whitmore, Dept Head *Chair's #: (860) 566-1867*	500 Brookfield St Hartford	06106				TCH	PBL			Publication withheld			
050	Bullard Havens Reg Voc-Tech Sch Miss Rita M Lambert, Dept Head *Chair's #: (203) 579-6117*	500 Palisades Ave Bridgeport	06610	2			TCH	PBL	12	12	43	54	39	0
051	E C Goodwin Reg Voc-Tech Sch Mrs Maureen Rabito, Dept Head *Chair's #: (860) 827-7731*	735 Slater Rd New Britain	06053				TCH	PBL	12	12	36	40	36	0
055	Eli Whitney Reg Voc-Tech Sch Mrs Joan T Novarro, Dept Head *Chair's #: (203) 397-4035*	71 Jones Rd Hamden	06514				TCH	PBL	12	12	32	41	24	0
058	Henry Abbott Reg Voc-Tech Sch Mrs Pamela P Cramer, Dept Head *Chair's #: (203) 797-2724*	Hayestown Rd Danbury	06810				TCH	PVT			Publication withheld			

School Code	Name of School, Director of Program, and Phone Number	Street Address / City or Town and Zip Code	Footnotes	Type of Program	NLNAC Accreditation as of January 31, 1999	Administrative Control	Financial Support (principal source)	Number of Months in Program	Educational Requirements for Entering Adult Program	Enrollments as of October 15, 1998	Admissions Aug. 1, 1997 - July 31, 1998	Graduations Aug. 1, 1997 - July 31, 1998	Fall Admissions Aug. 1, 1998 - Dec. 31, 1998
	CONNECTICUT												
	- Continued												
052	Howell Cheney Voc-Tech Sch / Ms Barbara Lindner, Dept Head / *Chair's #: (860) 253-3191*	791 W Middle Tpke / Manchester 06040				TCH	PBL			Publication withheld			
010	J M Wright Reg Voc-Tech Sch / Mrs Mimi Wright Maher, Head / *Chair's #: (203) 324-7363 Ext 33*	Scalzi Pk / Stamford 06904	2			TCH	PBL	0	12	24	32	17	32
057	Kaynor Reg Voc-Tech Sch / Mrs Judy Leonardi, Dept Head / *Chair's #: (203) 596-4302 Ext 33*	43 Tomkins St / Waterbury 06708	2			TCH	PBL	13	12	40	40	38	0
023	New England Technical Inst / Miss Eleanor Davio, Manager / *Chair's #: (860) 522-2261 Ext 148*	200 John Downey Dr / New Britain 06051				IND	PVT			Publication withheld			
011	Norwich Reg Voc-Tech Sch / Mrs Karen McKenney, Head / *Chair's #: (860) 859-5330*	590 New London Tpke / Norwich 06360				TCH	PBL	15	12	37	40	30	0
059	Vinal Reg Voc-Tech Sch / Mrs Margaret Andrews, Dept Head / *Chair's #: (860) 344-7141*	60 Daniels St / Middletown 06457				TCH	PBL	15	12	30	30	22	0
056	Windham Reg Voc-Tech Sch / Ms Maryann Donovan, Dept Head / *Chair's #: (860) 456-3879 Ext 156*	210 Birch St / Willimantic 06226				TCH	PBL			Publication withheld			
	DELAWARE												
	5 Programs in 4 Schools												
005	DE Tech & Comm Coll-Owens Campus / Mrs June Turansky, Chair / *Chair's #: (302) 856-1614*	PO Box 610 / Georgetown 19947				CC	PBL	11		23	25	18	23
004	DE Tech & Comm College-Terry Camp / Ms Ruth Yanos, Chair / *Chair's #: (302) 741-2924*	1832 N Dupont Pkwy / Dover 19901				CC	PBL	12	12	31	32	29	32
012	Delcastle Voc-Tech HS / Mrs Janet West, Director / *Chair's #: (302) 995-5619*	1417 Newport Rd / Wilmington 19804	HS			TCH	PBL	12	12	20	20	20	0
						TCH	PBL		12	54	18	16	18
	DISTRICT OF COLUMBIA												
	3 Programs in 3 Schools												
004	Harrison Center For Career Educ / Mrs Arthuretta Zeigler, Dir / *Chair's #: (202) 628-5672 Ext 308*	624 9th St NW / Washington 20007			A	IND	PVT	12	12	67	74	42	28
005	Health Management Inc / Ms Eleanor Browning, Exec Dir / *Chair's #: (202) 291-9020*	6856 Eastern Ave NW 376 / Washington 20012				IND	PVT			Publication withheld			

Explanation of footnotes on page x

School Code	Name of School, Director of Program, and Phone Number	Street Address / City or Town and Zip Code	Footnotes	Type of Program	NLNAC Accreditation as of January 31, 1999	Administrative Control	Financial Support (principal source)	Number of Months in Program	Educational Requirements for Entering Adult Program	Enrollments as of October 15, 1998	Admissions Aug. 1, 1997 - July 31, 1998	Graduations Aug. 1, 1997 - July 31, 1998	Fall Admissions Aug. 1, 1998 - Dec. 31, 1998
	DISTRICT OF COLUMBIA **- Continued**												
003	Margaret Murray Washington Voc HS Dr Ruth Richardson, Coord *Chair's #: (202) 673-7436 Ext 202*	27 O St NW Washington 20001			A	TCH	PBL			Publication withheld			
	FLORIDA **44 Programs in 44 Schools**												
013	Academy For Practical Nursing Hlth Oc Mrs Lois Gackenheimer, Dir *Chair's #: (561) 683-1400*	5154 Okeechobee Blvd Suite 2 West Palm Beach 33417	2			COL	PVT	10	12	43	45	44	0
002	Allied Hlth Training Center Inc Ms Beverly Pryce, Dir *Chair's #: (954) 961-9466*	4350 W Hallandale Hollywood 33023	2			TCH	PVT			Publication withheld			
038	Brevard Comm College Ms Constance Bobik, Chair *Chair's #: (407) 632-1111*	1519 Clearlake Rd Cocoa 32922				CC	PBL			21	24	21	0
024	Broward Co Pract Nsg Progs (4 Centers) Ms Barbara L Zygowsky, Specialist *Chair's #: (954) 760-7409*	600 SE 3rd Ave Fort Lauderdale 33301	 HS HSE		A A A	TCH TCH TCH	PBL PBL PBL		 12	Publication withheld			
053	Central Florida Comm College Dr Lapham-Alcorn, Assoc Dean *Chair's #: (352) 237-2111 Ext 1275*	3001 SW College Rd Ocala 32674			A	CC	PBL	12	12	27	36	29	0
044	Charlotte Co Voc-Tech Ctr Mrs Yvonne B Meinket, Supervisor *Chair's #: (941) 629-6819 Ext 136*	18300 Toledo Blade Blvd Port Charlotte 33948				TCH	PBL			Publication withheld			
022	Chipola Jr College Ms Kathy Wheeler, Dir *Chair's #: (850) 718-2278*	3094 Indian Circle Marianna 32466				CC	PBL	12	12	20	24	21	0
007	Dade Co Public Schs (4 Centers) Ms Rose Hodge, Chair *Chair's #: (305) 995-2827*	1450 NE 2nd Ave Rm 816 Miami 33132			A	TCH	PBL			Publication withheld			
020	Daytona Beach Comm College Ms Barbara Doyle, Chair *Chair's #: (904) 255-8131 Ext 3720*	1200 Volusia Ave Box 2811 Daytona Beach 32120				CC	PBL	11	11	83	96	56	36
047	Desoto County PN Prog Ms Janet Loporto, Instructor *Chair's #: (941) 494-4222 Ext 148*	530 La Solono Ave Arcadia 33821				SEC	PBL	12	12	12	12	10	12
031	Florida Comm College at Jacksonville Dr June Chandler, Dir *Chair's #: (904) 766-6592*	4501 Capper Rd Campus C212 Jacksonville 32218	7			CC	PBL	10	12	0	0	70	0

School Code	Name of School, Director of Program, and Phone Number	Street Address / City or Town and Zip Code	Footnotes	Type of Program	NLNAC Accreditation as of January 31, 1999	Administrative Control	Financial Support (principal source)	Number of Months in Program	Educational Requirements for Entering Adult Program	Enrollments as of October 15, 1998	Admissions Aug. 1, 1997 - July 31, 1998	Graduations Aug. 1, 1997 - July 31, 1998	Fall Admissions Aug. 1, 1998 - Dec. 31, 1998
	FLORIDA												
	- Continued												
026	Florida Hosp College of Hlth Sciences Ms Victoria Hughes, Chair *Chair's #: (407) 895-7893 Ext 1083*	795 Lake Estelle Dr Orlando 32803				CC	PVT	11	12	37	40	34	39
015	Gadsden Tech Inst Ms Glenda Battle, Coord *Chair's #: (850) 875-8324 Ext 129*	201 Martin Luther King Blvd Quincy 32351	2			TCH	PBL	12	12	19	17	12	19
006	Hillsborough Co-Erwin V-T Ctr Mrs Cheryl Brown, Dept Head *Chair's #: (813) 231-1800 Ext 2447*	2010 E Hillsborough Ave Tampa 33610				TCH	PBL	12	12	191	233	166	97
004	Hlth Inst of Tampa Bay Ms Sharon A Roberts, Dir *Chair's #: (813) 577-1497*	9549 Koger Blvd Suite 100 St Petersburg 33702				IND	PVT			Publication withheld			
033	Indian River Comm College Ms Jane P Cebelak, Director *Chair's #: (561) 462-4778*	3209 Virginia Ave Fort Pierce 34981				CC	PBL	12	11	77	50	55	48
035	James L Walker Tech Ctr Mrs Sally Holland, Coord *Chair's #: (941) 643-0919 Ext 6655*	3702 Estey Ave, N Naples 34104				TCH	PBL	12	12	70	72	55	48
057	Lake City Comm College Mrs Judy Clemons, Coord *Chair's #: (904) 752-1822 Ext 1150*	Route 19 Box 1030 Lake City 32025				CC	PBL	12	12	25	24	20	0
032	Lake County Area Voc-Tech Ctr Ms Elaine Rejimbal, Chair *Chair's #: (352) 742-6497 Ext 134*	2001 Kurt St Eustis 32726				TCH	PBL	11	12	48	56	41	31
029	Lee County Sch of PN Mrs Sheila Sarver, Dir *Chair's #: (941) 334-4544 Ext 0342*	3800 Michigan Ave Fort Myers 33916				TCH	PBL	12	11	56	77	52	23
011	Lively Tech Ctr Ms Judith G Hankin, Dir *Chair's #: (904) 487-7452*	500 N Appleyard Dr Tallahassee 32304				TCH	PBL			Publication withheld			
027	Manatee Tech Inst Mrs Faith Herring, Chair *Chair's #: (941) 751-7957*	5603 34th St West Bradenton 34210				TCH	PBL	12	12	53	88	55	31
045	Mercy Hospital Mr James Bray, Dir *Chair's #: (305) 285-2777*	3663 S Miami Ave Miami 33133			A	HSP	PVT	11	12	42	40	31	45
021	North Florida Comm Coll Mr Karen Steward, Coord *Chair's #: (850) 973-2288 Ext 134*	1000 Turner Davis Dr Madison 32340				CC	PBL			Publication withheld			

Explanation of footnotes on page x

FLORIDA

- Continued

School Code	Name of School, Director of Program, and Phone Number	Street Address / City or Town and Zip Code	Footnotes	Type of Program	NLNAC Accreditation as of January 31, 1999	Administrative Control	Financial Support (principal source)	Number of Months in Program	Educational Requirements for Entering Adult Program	Enrollments as of October 15, 1998	Admissions Aug. 1, 1997 - July 31, 1998	Graduations Aug. 1, 1997 - July 31, 1998	Fall Admissions Aug. 1, 1998 - Dec. 31, 1998
005	Okaloosa Applied Tech Center Mrs Sylvia Austin, Dept Head *Chair's #: (904)-833-3500 Ext 3544*	1976 Lewis Turner Blvd Ft Walton Beach 32547				TCH	PBL			53	60	48	0
023	OrangeTech Ed Ctr-Orlando Tech Mrs Yvonne Julien, Chair *Chair's #: (407) 317-3371*	301 W Amelia St Orlando 32801				TCH	PBL	12	12	110	146	72	50
025	Palm Beach Co PN Program (3 Centers) Mrs Donna Jordan, Specialist *Chair's #: (561) 434-7467*	3312 Forest Hill Blvd #A330 West Palm Beach 33406				TCH	PBL	15	12	121	128	81	62
046	Pasco-Hernando Comm College Ms Karen Richardson, Dir *Chair's #: (727) 816-3280*	10230 Ridge Rd New Port Richey 34654				CC	PBL	11	12	56	72	56	36
003	Pensacola Jr College Dr Joan Connell, Dept Head *Chair's #: (850) 484-2254*	5555 W Hwy 98 Pensacola 32507				CC	PBL			82	94	43	0
009	Pinellas Tech Educ Center Mrs Evelyn Gardner, Chair *Chair's #: (727) 893-2500 Ext 1071*	901 34th St, S St Petersburg 33711				TCH	PBL			106	139	96	87
016	Pinellas Tech Educ Ctr Mrs Candace Gioia, Chair *Chair's #: (727) 538-7167 Ext 1128*	6100 154th Ave, N Clearwater 34620				TCH	PBL			Publication withheld			
059	Port St Lucie Sch of PN Ms Mabel Smith-Duffus, Dir *Chair's #: (561) 398-0102*	10792 South Federal Highway Port St Lucie 34952				TCH	PBL			Publication withheld			
014	Santa Fe Comm College Ms Rita Sutherland, Dir *Chair's #: (352) 395-5703 Ext 5737*	3000 NW 83rd St W-201 Gainesville 32606	A			CC	PBL	11	12	30	30	25	30
017	Sarasota Co Vocational Tech Inst Dr Linda Swisher, Chair *Chair's #: (941) 924-1365 Ext 372*	4748 Beneva Rd Sarasota 34233	A			TCH	PBL	12	12	72	77	40	41
030	Seminole Comm College Ms Sharon Cannon, Manager *Chair's #: (407) 328-2018*	100 Weldon Blvd Sanford 32773				CC	PBL	12	12	50	58	42	0
042	South Florida Comm College Dr Mary Ann Fritz, Chair *Chair's #: (941) 453-6661 Ext 118*	600 W College Dr Avon Park 33825				CC	PBL			19	23	19	20
028	St Augustine Tech Ctr Mrs Nancy Lee Thomas, Manager *Chair's #: (904) 823-1383 Ext 1383*	2980 Collins Avenue St Augustine 32095				TCH	PBL	12	12	49	48	38	24

Explanation of footnotes on page x

School Code	Name of School, Director of Program, and Phone Number	Street Address / City or Town and Zip Code	Footnotes	Type of Program	NLNAC Accreditation as of January 31, 1999	Administrative Control	Financial Support (principal source)	Number of Months in Program	Educational Requirements for Entering Adult Program	Enrollments as of October 15, 1998	Admissions Aug. 1, 1997 - July 31, 1998	Graduations Aug. 1, 1997 - July 31, 1998	Fall Admissions Aug. 1, 1998 - Dec. 31, 1998
	FLORIDA												
	- Continued												
037	Suwannee-Hamilton Area Vo-Tech Ctr Mrs Virginia Stebbins, Director *Chair's #: (904) 364-2784 Ext 2784*	415 SW Pinewood Dr Live Oak 32060				TCH	PBL			18	20	14	20
061	Technical Education Center Ms Karen Guritz, Director *Chair's #: (407) 344-5080 Ext 128*	501 Simpson Rd Kissimmee 34744				TCH	PBL			Publication withheld			
019	Tom P Haney Tech Center Ms Lanita Hill, Director *Chair's #: (850) 747-5500 Ext 111*	3016 Hwy 77 Panama City 32405				TCH	PBL			Publication withheld			
010	Traviss Tech Center Ms JoAnn Hagghloom, Dir *Chair's #: (941) 499-2700 Ext 2715*	3225 Winter Lake Rd Lakeland 33803				TCH	PBL			94	96	71	95
039	Washington-Holmes Tech Center Ms Patricia Cordell, Coord *Chair's #: (850) 638-1180 Ext 351*	209 Hoyt St Chipley 32428				TCH	PBL			Publication withheld			
043	Withlacoochee Tech Inst Mrs Jan Lesight, Coord *Chair's #: (352) 726-2430 Ext 233*	1201 W Main St Inverness 34450				TCH	PBL			Publication withheld			
	GEORGIA												
	48 Programs in 43 Schools												
019	Albany Tech Institute Mrs Dorothy K Garner, Dir *Chair's #: (912) 430-3555*	1021 Lowe Rd Albany 31701				TCH	PBL	15	12	33	54	28	33
011	Altamaha Tech Inst Ms Susan Strickland, Chair *Chair's #: (912) 427-5803*	1777 W Cherry St Jesup 31545				TCH	PBL			Publication withheld			
026	Athens Area Tech Inst Mrs Joyce Manus, Dir *Chair's #: (706) 355-5058*	800 US Hwy 29 N Athens 30610				TCH	PBL	15	12	24	40	21	40
013	Atlanta Tech Inst Ms Patricia Blake, Chair *Chair's #: (404) 756-3719*	1560 Metropolitan Pkwy Atlanta 30310				TCH	PBL			Publication withheld			
050	Augusta Tech Institute (2 Divs) Mrs Sara Youngblood, Dept Head *Chair's #: (706) 771-4190*	3116 Deans Bridge Rd Augusta 30906			A	TCH	PBL	15	12	151	119	47	50
020	Bainbridge College Ms Lisa Sharber, Chair *Chair's #: (912) 248-2530*	2500 E Shotwell St Bainbridge 31717				CC	PBL			Publication withheld			

Explanation of footnotes on page x

School Code	Name of School, Director of Program, and Phone Number	Street Address, City or Town and Zip Code	Footnotes	Type of Program	NLNAC Accreditation as of January 31, 1999	Administrative Control	Financial Support (principal source)	Number of Months in Program	Educational Requirements for Entering Adult Program	Enrollments as of October 15, 1998	Admissions Aug. 1, 1997 - July 31, 1998	Graduations Aug. 1, 1997 - July 31, 1998	Fall Admissions Aug. 1, 1998 - Dec. 31, 1998
	GEORGIA **- Continued**												
032	Carroll Tech Inst Ms Cheryl Hooks, Chair *Chair's #: (770) 836-6800*	997 So Hwy-16 Carrollton 30116				TCH	PBL			Publication withheld			
038	Chattahoochee Tech Institute (2 Divs) Mrs Marilyn Mintz, Chair *Chair's #: (770) 528-4568*	980 S Cobb Dr SE Marietta 30060				TCH	PBL	15	12	38	40	22	41
036	Coastal GA Comm Coll Mrs Kay Hampton, Chair *Chair's #: (912) 262-3340*	3700 Altama Ave Brunswick 31522				CC	PBL	15	12	25	35	28	25
074	Columbus Tech Institute Dr Margaret Gursel, Dept Head *Chair's #: (706) 649-1840*	928 45th St Columbus 31904				TCH	PBL			Publication withheld			
007	Coosa Valley Tech Institute Dr Dolores Linatoc, Chair *Chair's #: (706) 297-6963*	785 Cedar Ave Rome 30161				TCH	PBL			Publication withheld			
024	Dalton Coll-PN Prog Mrs Carolyn Higgins, Coord *Chair's #: (706) 278-8922*	1221 Elkwood Dr Dalton 30720				TCH	PBL	16	12	18	46	21	15
037	DeKalb Tech Institute (2 Divs) Ms Geri Moreland, Dept Chair *Chair's #: (404) 297-9522 Ext 1128*	495 N Indian Creek Dr Clarkston 30021				TCH	PBL			Publication withheld			
072	East Central Tech Institute (2 Divs) Ms Faye Elliott, Lead Instructor *Chair's #: (912) 468-7487 Ext 2108*	PO Box 1069 667 Perry House Fitzgerald 31750				TCH	PBL			Publication withheld			
040	Flint River Tech Inst (2 Divs) Mrs F McDowell, Lead Instructor *Chair's #: (706) 646-6185 Ext 6181*	Box 1089 US Hwy 19 South Thomaston 30286				TCH	PBL			Publication withheld			
017	Griffin Technical Inst Ms Joyce Hickey, Dept Head *Chair's #: (770) 228-7348*	501 Varsity Rd Griffin 30223	2			TCH	PBL			24	41	21	20
091	Gwinnett Tech Inst Ms Cathy Kelley, Dir *Chair's #: (404) 962-7580 Ext 178*	5150 Sugarloaf Parkway Lawrenceville 30246				TCH	PBL			Publication withheld			
097	Heart of GA Tech Inst (2 Branches) Mrs June Williams, Chair *Chair's #: (912) 374-7122*	560 Pinehill Rd Dublin 31021				TCH	PBL			Publication withheld			
084	Lanier Tech Institute Mrs Gail Adam, Instructor *Chair's #: (404) 531-6300 Ext 6371*	PO Box 58 2990 Landrum Edu Oakwood 30566				TCH	PBL			Publication withheld			

Explanation of footnotes on page x

School Code	Name of School, Director of Program, and Phone Number	Street Address, City or Town and Zip Code	Footnotes	Type of Program	NLNAC Accreditation as of January 31, 1999	Administrative Control	Financial Support (principal source)	Number of Months in Program	Educational Requirements for Entering Adult Program	Enrollments as of October 15, 1998	Admissions Aug. 1, 1997 - July 31, 1998	Graduations Aug. 1, 1997 - July 31, 1998	Fall Admissions Aug. 1, 1998 - Dec. 31, 1998
	GEORGIA												
	- Continued												
043	Macon Tech Baldwin County Ms Sue Hodell, Chair *Chair's #: (912) 445-2330*	PO Box 1009 Hwy 49 W Milledgeville 31061				TCH	PBL			Publication withheld			
009	Macon Tech Institute (2 Divs) Mrs Teresa Wilkins, Head *Chair's #: (912) 757-3585*	3300 Macon Tech Dr Macon 31206				TCH	PBL	15	12	60	76	47	18
083	Middle GA Tech Institute Ms Julia Nell Shaw, Director *Chair's #: (912) 988-6800 Ext 130*	80 Corten Walker, Dr Warner Robins 31088				TCH	PBL			Publication withheld			
066	Moultrie Area Tech Inst (2 Divs) Ms Debra Craft, Chair *Chair's #: (912) 891-7000*	361 Industrial Dr Moultrie 31768				TCH	PBL			Publication withheld			
015	North Georgia Tech Inst (2 Branches) Mrs Melinda Shiflet, Instructor *Chair's #: (706) 754-7762*	GA Hwy 197 N Po Box 65 Clarkesville 30523				TCH	PBL	15	12	49	60	49	25
090	North Western Tech Inst Mrs Pat Caldwell, Coord *Chair's #: (706) 764-3716*	265 Bicentennial Trail Rock Spring 30739				CC	PBL	15	12	52	50	0	52
903	Ogeechee Tech Inst Mrs Carol Turknett, Instructor *Chair's #: (912) 871-1627*	One Joe Kennedy Blvd Statesboro 30458				TCH	PBL			Publication withheld			
010	Okefenokee Tech Inst Ms Willene Griffin Fox, Dir *Chair's #: (912) 287-5836*	1701 Carswell Ave Waycross 31503				TCH	PBL			Publication withheld			
065	Pickens Tech Inst Ms Patricia Turner, Instructor *Chair's #: (706) 692-4500*	100 Pickens Tech Dr Jasper 30143				TCH	PBL	15	12	53	92	39	24
001	Sauderville Reg Tech Inst Ms Kathy Claxton, Coord *Chair's #: ((912) 553-2088*	1189 Deepsted Rd Box 6179 Sandersville 31082	2			TCH	PBL			Publication withheld			
008	Savannah Tech Sch (2 Branches) Mrs Victoria Agyekum, Dept Head *Chair's #: (912) 553-2088*	5717 White Bluff Rd Savannah 31405			A	TCH	PBL	15	12	76	60	55	40
002	South Georgia Tech Inst (2 Branches) Mrs Joyce Dunmon, Chair *Chair's #: (912) 931-2004*	1583 Southerfield Rd Americus 31709				TCH	PBL			Publication withheld			
901	Southeastern Tech Inst (2 Branches) Mrs Linda Grancen, Instructor *Chair's #: (912) 538-3144 Ext 3002*	3001 E First St Vidalia 30474				TCH	PBL			Publication withheld			

Explanation of footnotes on page x

School Code	Name of School, Director of Program, and Phone Number	Street Address / City or Town and Zip Code		Footnotes	Type of Program	NLNAC Accreditation as of January 31, 1999	Administrative Control	Financial Support (principal source)	Number of Months in Program	Educational Requirements for Entering Adult Program	Enrollments as of October 15, 1998	Admissions Aug. 1, 1997 - July 31, 1998	Graduations Aug. 1, 1997 - July 31, 1998	Fall Admissions Aug. 1, 1998 - Dec. 31, 1998
	GEORGIA													
	- Continued													
039	Swainsboro Tech Inst / Ms Janice Black, Coord / *Chair's #: (912) 289-2200*	346 Kite Rd / Swainsboro	30401				TCH	PBL			Publication withheld			
041	Thomas Tech Inst / Dr Annie McElroy, Dept Head / *Chair's #: (912) 225-5200*	15689 US Hwy 19 N / Thomasville	31792				TCH	PBL	18	12	38	23	14	21
052	Tift Sch of PN (Div of Moultrie) / Ms Wanda Golden, Dir / *Chair's #: (912) 382-2767*	302 E 14th St / Tifton	31794				TCH	PBL			Publication withheld			
022	Valdosta Tech Inst / Mrs Jackie Sorrell, Chair / *Chair's #: (912) 333-2110*	4089 Val -Tech Rd Box 928 / Valdosta	31603				TCH	PBL			43	70	24	35
012	West Georgia Tech Inst / Ms Beverly Cochran, Dir / *Chair's #: (706) 845-4323 Ext 5729*	303 Fort Dr / La Grange	30240				TCH	PBL			23	24	17	12
	HAWAII													
	4 Programs in 4 Schools													
002	Hawaii Comm College / Dr Elizabeth Ojala, Dir / *Chair's #: (808) 974-7560*	Hilo	96720				CC	PBL			Publication withheld			
001	Kapiolani Comm College / Mrs Joan Matsukawa, Chair / *Chair's #: (807) 734-9301*	4303 Diamond Head Rd / Honolulu	96814				CC	PBL			Publication withheld			
004	Kauai Comm College / Mr Richard Carmichael, Dir / *Chair's #: (808) 245-8255*	3-1901 Kaumualii Hwy / Lihue Kauai	96766				CC	PBL	12	12	23	24	16	24
005	Maui Comm College-Career Ladder / Mrs Nancy Johnson, Chair / *Chair's #: (808) 984-3250*	310 Kaahumanu Ave / Kahului Maui	96732				CC	PBL			65	41	57	0
	IDAHO													
	5 Programs in 5 Schools													
026	Boise State Univ-Dept of Nsg / Mrs Mary A Towle, Dir / *Chair's #: (208) 426-3845*	1910 Univ Dr / Boise	83725				CC	PBL	11	12	42	50	33	20
024	Coll of So Idaho Voc-Tech Sch / Dr Claudeen R Buettner, Chair / *Chair's #: (208) 733-9554 Ext 2155*	PO Box 1238 / Twin Falls	83303				TCH	PBL	11	12	30	30	25	20
046	Eastern Idaho Tech College / Ms Kathleen Nelson, Manager / *Chair's #: (208) 524-3000 Ext 3340*	1600 S 25th / Idaho Falls	83404				TCH	PBL			Publication withheld			

School Code	Name of School, Director of Program, and Phone Number	Street Address / City or Town and Zip Code		Footnotes	Type of Program	NLNAC Accreditation as of January 31, 1999	Administrative Control	Financial Support (principal source)	Number of Months in Program	Educational Requirements for Entering Adult Program	Enrollments as of October 15, 1998	Admissions Aug. 1, 1997 - July 31, 1998	Graduations Aug. 1, 1997 - July 31, 1998	Fall Admissions Aug. 1, 1998 - Dec. 31, 1998
	IDAHO													
	- Continued													
030	Idaho State Univ-Sch of Applied Tech Ms Suzanne Griffin-Lawson, Chair *Chair's #: (208) 236-2507 Ext 2507*	Box 8380 Pocatello	83209				TCH	PBL			Publication withheld			
043	North Idaho College Voc-Tech Sch Mrs Joan Brogan, Dir *Chair's #: (208) 769-3480*	W 1000 Garden Ave Coeur D'Alene	83814	7			TCH	PBL			Data reported w/AD prog			
	ILLINOIS													
	40 Programs in 37 Schools													
056	Beck Area Voc Ctr Ms Janice Augustine, Director *Chair's #: (618) 473-2222*	6137 Beck Rd Red Bud	62278				TCH	PBL	11	12	38	68	54	22
028	Black Hawk College Dr Sally Flesch, Chair *Chair's #: (309) 796-1311 Ext 3153*	6600 34th Ave Moline	61265				CC	PBL	9	12	24	41	31	24
052	Capital Area Sch of PN Ms Jamie Hamilton, Coord *Chair's #: (217) 585-2162*	2201 Toronto Rd Springfield	62707			A	TCH	PBL	11	12	108	87	72	60
029	Carl Sandburg College Ms Alice Enderlin, Coord *Chair's #: (309) 341-5253*	2232 S Lake Storey Rd Galesburg	61401				CC	PBL	10	12	31	27	16	36
011	Chicago Public Schools Ms Sandra Webb, Coord *Chair's #: (773) 534-7890*	2045 W Jackson Chicago	60612		HS HSE	A A A	SEC SEC SEC	PBL PBL PBL		11	Publication withheld			
034	City College of Chi-Hlth Occup Careers Mrs M Ward-Ellison, Dir *Chair's #: (773) 451-2000 Ext 2016*	3901 S State Chicago	60609				TCH	PBL			Publication withheld			
001	City Colleges of Chicago-W Wright Coll Ms Ingrid Forsberg, Dir *Chair's #: (773) 489-8915*	1645 N California Chicago	60647				CC	PBL	11	12	51	31	36	36
025	Danville Area Comm College Mrs Ann Wagle, Dir *Chair's #: (217) 443-8814*	2000 E Main St Danville	61832				CC	PBL			Publication withheld			
004	Decatur School of PN-Area Voc Ctr Mrs Mary L Cookson, Dir *Chair's #: (217) 424-3075*	300 E Eldorado St Decatur	62523				TCH	PBL	12	12	42	47	26	28
057	Elgin Comm College Mrs Maryann Vaca, Assoc Dean *Chair's #: (847) 888-7350*	1700 Spartan Dr Elgin	60123	7			CC	PBL			Data reported w/AD Prog			

Explanation of footnotes on page x

School Code	Name of School, Director of Program, and Phone Number	Street Address / City or Town and Zip Code		Footnotes	Type of Program	NLNAC Accreditation as of January 31, 1999	Administrative Control	Financial Support (principal source)	Number of Months in Program	Educational Requirements for Entering Adult Program	Enrollments as of October 15, 1998	Admissions Aug. 1, 1997 - July 31, 1998	Graduations Aug. 1, 1997 - July 31, 1998	Fall Admissions Aug. 1, 1998 - Dec. 31, 1998
	ILLINOIS													
	- Continued													
003	F W Olin Voc School-Alton PN Prog; Mrs Joann Peuterbaugh, Coord; Chair's #: (618) 463-2092	4200 Humbert Rd; Alton	62002				TCH	PBL	11	12	18	26	16	12
060	Heartland Comm College; Ms Jacqueline Perley, Dir; Chair's #: (309) 827-0500 Ext 448	1226 Towanda Ave; Bloomington	61701	7			CC	PBL			Data reported w/AD Prog			
049	Highland Comm College; Mrs Alice Nied, Dir; Chair's #: (815) 235-6121 Ext 315	2998 Pearl City Rd; Freeport	61032				CC	PBL			Publication withheld			
053	IL Eastern Comm Colleges Dist 529; Dr Judy Johnson, Assoc Dean; Chair's #: (618) 395-7777 Ext 2136	305 North West St; Olney	62450				CC	PBL	11	12	138	140	96	140
044	Illinois Central College; Ms Mary Beth Kiefner, Supv; Chair's #: (309) 999-4600	201 SW Adams; East Peoria	61635			A	CC	PBL			Publication withheld			
051	Illinois Valley Comm College; Mrs Bonnie Grusk, Chair; Chair's #: (815) 224-2720 Ext 485	815 Orlando Smith Ave; Oglesby	61348				CC	PBL	11	12	19	17	27	20
048	John A Logan College; Mrs Debra Goddard, Dir; Chair's #: (618) 985-2828 Ext 8455	700 Logan College Rd; Carterville	62918				CC	PBL	12		89	70	67	67
022	John Wood Comm College-PN; Mrs Julie Barry, Dir; Chair's #: (217) 224-6564 Ext 4544	150 S 48th St; Quincy	62301				CC	PBL	12	12	32	46	40	0
031	Joliet Township HS; Mrs Arthetta Reeder, Dir; Chair's #: (815) 727-6885	201 E Jefferson; Joliet	60432				TCH	PBL	11	12	34	66	46	44
033	Kankakee Comm College; Mrs Phyllis Nichols, Director; Chair's #: (815) 933-0295	Box 888 River Dr; Kankakee	60901				CC	PBL			Publication withheld			
055	Kaskaskia College; Mrs Marylou Whitten, Dir; Chair's #: (618) 532-1981 Ext 226	27210 College Rd; Centralia	62801				CC	PBL	11	12	35	28	20	22
042	Kishwaukee College-PN Sch; Ms Heather Peters, Dir; Chair's #: (815) 825-2086 Ext 355	21193 Malta Rd; Malta	60150	7			CC	PBL			Data reported w/AD Prog			
016	Lake Land College; Kathleen Doehring, Dir; Chair's #: (217) 234-5204	5001 Lake Land Blvd; Mattoon	61938			A	CC	PBL	12	12	38	36	27	40

School Code	Name of School, Director of Program, and Phone Number	Street Address City or Town and Zip Code		Footnotes	Type of Program	NLNAC Accreditation as of January 31, 1999	Administrative Control	Financial Support (principal source)	Number of Months in Program	Educational Requirements for Entering Adult Program	Enrollments as of October 15, 1998	Admissions Aug. 1, 1997 - July 31, 1998	Graduators Aug. 1, 1997 - July 31, 1998	Fall Admissions Aug. 1, 1998 - Dec. 31, 1998
	ILLINOIS													
	- Continued													
061	Lewis and Clark Comm Coll Dr Linda Smith, Coord *Chair's #: (618) 466-3411 Ext 4431*	5800 Godfrey Rd Godfrey	62035				CC	PBL	12	12	14	13	9	18
006	Lincolnland Comm College Ms Joan Lewis, Dept Chair *Chair's #: (217) 786-2200*	5250 Shephard Rd Springfield	62794				CC	PBL			Publication withheld			
059	Morton College Mrs Aline Tupa, Coord *Chair's #: (708) 656-8000*	3801 South Central Ave Cicero	60804	7			CC	PBL			Data reported w/AD prog			
047	Oakton Comm College Ms Marilou Wasseluk, Chair *Chair's #: (847) 635-1720*	1600 East Golf Road Des Plaines	60016	7			CC	PBL			Data reported w/AD prog			
050	Parkland College-PN prog Dr Sharon A Gerth, Chair *Chair's #: (217) 351-2289*	2400 W Bradley Ave Champaign	61821	7		A	CC	PBL			Data reported w/AD prog			
023	Rend Lake College Ms Wilanna Patton, Chair *Chair's #: (618) 437-5321 Ext 225*	Ina	62846				CC	PBL			Publication withheld			
019	Rockford School of Practical Nursing Mrs S Carlson Asher, Dir *Chair's #: (815) 966-3714*	978 Haskell Ave Rockford	61103			A	SEC	PBL	11	12	24	31	24	24
026	Sauk Valley Comm Coll Ms Rosemary Johnson, Director *Chair's #: (815) 288-5511 Ext 376*	173 Illinois Route #2 Dixon	61021				CC	PBL			Publication withheld			
043	Shawnee Comm College Dr Jeannine Hayduk, Dir *Chair's #: (618) 634-2242 Ext 200*	8364 Shawnee College Rd Ullin	62992				CC	PBL			Publication withheld			
046	South Suburban College Ms Judith A Coglianese, Exec Dir *Chair's #: (708) 596-2000 Ext 2260*	15800 S State St South Holland	60473			A	CC	PBL	11	12	49	47	23	50
012	Southeastern Illinois College Mrs Nancy Buttry, Dir *Chair's #: (618) 252-5400 Ext 2331*	3575 College Rd Harrisburg	62946				CC	PBL			Publication withheld			
045	Spoon River College Dr Janis Waite, Assoc Dean *Chair's #: (309) 649-6333*	23235 N County 22 Canton	61520	7			CC	PBL			Data Reported w/AD Prog			
039	Triton College Mrs Sharon Abbate, Chair *Chair's #: (708) 456-0300 Ext 3656*	2000 5th Ave River Grove	60171			A	CC	PBL	12	12	89	92	84	53

School Code	Name of School, Director of Program, and Phone Number	Street Address / City or Town and Zip Code	Footnotes	Type of Program	NLNAC Accreditation as of January 31, 1999	Administrative Control	Financial Support (principal source)	Number of Months in Program	Educational Requirements for Entering Adult Program	Enrollments as of October 15, 1998	Admissions Aug. 1, 1997 - July 31, 1998	Graduations Aug. 1, 1997 - July 31, 1998	Fall Admissions Aug. 1, 1998 - Dec. 31, 1998
	ILLINOIS												
	- Continued												
041	William Rainey Harper College Mrs Cheryl Wandambi, Dir *Chair's #: (847) 925-6533*	1200 West Algonquin Rd Palatine 60067	7			CC	PBL			Data reported w/AD prog			
	INDIANA												
	23 Programs in 23 Schools												
016	Anderson PN Sch-Anderson Comm Schs Mrs Marcia Scott, Dir *Chair's #: (765) 683-3015*	325 W 38th St Anderson 46013				TCH	PBL	12	12	27	32	30	16
031	Horizon Career College Ms Cristine Pytel, Coord *Chair's #: (219) 756-6811*	8315 Virginia St Suite A Merrillville 46410				CC	PBL			Publication withheld			
020	Indiana V-T College Sch of PN, Reg 1 Mrs Gene Ann Shapinsky, Chair *Chair's #: (812) 265-2580 Ext 4167*	Hwy 62 & Ivy Tech Dr Madison 47250				TCH	PBL			Publication withheld			
018	Indiana V-T College Sch of PN, Reg 1 Mrs Karen Warner, Chair *Chair's #: (219) 464-8514 Ext 225*	2401 Valley Dr Valparaiso 46383	A			TCH	PBL	12	12	109	85	79	65
013	Indiana V-T College Sch of PN, Reg 10 Ms Celinda K Leach, Chair *Chair's #: (812) 332-1559 Ext 4325*	3116 Canterbury Ct Bloomington 47402				TCH	PBL	12	12	62	82	44	43
005	Indiana V-T College Sch of PN, Reg 2 Ms Beth Krakowski, Chair *Chair's #: (219) 236-7173 Ext 720*	1534 W Sample St South Bend 46619				TCH	PBL			Publication withheld			
008	Indiana V-T College Sch of PN, Reg 7 Mrs Leota Ehm, Chair *Chair's #: (812) 299-1121 Ext 287*	7999 US. Highway 41S. Terre Haute 47802				CC	PBL	12	12	104	109	70	48
002	Indiana V-T College Sch of PN, Reg 7 Mrs Lucy White, Chair *Chair's #: (765) 653-7410*	12 North Jackson Greencastle 46135				TCH	PBL	12	12	25	30	21	29
011	Indiana V-T College Sch of PN, Reg 9 Mrs Jillene Anderson, Chair *Chair's #: (765) 966-2656 Ext 374*	2325 Chester Blvd Richmond 47374				TCH	PBL	12	12	85	85	64	85
024	Indiana Voc Tech Coll Reg12 Mrs Elaine Schmidt, Chair *Chair's #: (812) 429-1904*	3501 First Ave Evansville 47710	A			TCH	PBL	12	12	48	48	38	49
017	IVTC , Reg 4 Mrs Marsha Duda, Chair *Chair's #: (765)-772-9199*	3208 Ross Rd PO Box 6299 Lafayette 47903				TCH	PBL	12	12	81	100	57	50

School Code	Name of School, Director of Program, and Phone Number	Street Address City or Town and Zip Code		Footnotes	Type of Program	NLNAC Accreditation as of January 31, 1999	Administrative Control	Financial Support (principal source)	Number of Months in Program	Educational Requirements for Entering Adult Program	Enrollments as of October 15, 1998	Admissions Aug. 1, 1997 - July 31, 1998	Graduations Aug. 1, 1997 - July 31, 1998	Fall Admissions Aug. 1, 1998 - Dec. 31, 1998
	INDIANA													
	- Continued													
009	IVY Tech State Coll -Hlth Tech State Co Ms Geneva Lamm, Chair *Chair's #: (812) 372-9925 Ext 134*	4475 Central Ave Columbus	47203				TCH	PBL	12	12	107	80	0	76
010	Ivy Tech State Coll Reg 13 Ms Sue Jewell, Chair *Chair's #: (812) 246-3301 Ext 4195*	8204 Hwy 311 Sellersburg	47172				TCH	PBL			Publication withheld			
006	IVY Tech State Coll Reg 3 Mrs JoAnn Dever, Chair *Chair's #: (219) 480-4272*	3800 N Anthony Blvd Fort Wayne	46805				TCH	PBL			Publication withheld			
900	IVY Tech State Coll Reg 6 Mrs Catherine Woodward, Chair *Chair's #: (765) 289-2291 Ext 341*	4301 South Cowan Rd Muncie	47302				CC	PBL			Publication withheld			
030	IVY Tech State Coll-Reg 5 Mrs Laurie Peters, Chair *Chair's #: (765) 459-0561 Ext 385*	1815 E Morgan Box 1373 Kokomo	46903				TCH	PBL	12	12	50	50	38	50
023	IVY Tech State College Reg 1 Ms Saundra Horne, Chair *Chair's #: (219) 981-1111*	1440 East 35th Ave Gary	46409				TCH	PBL			92	67	40	36
001	Ivy Tech State College Reg 8 Ms Barbara Deady, Chair *Chair's #: (317) 921-4407*	One West 26th St Box 1763 Indianapolis	46206			A	TCH	PBL	12	12	129	140	99	70
019	J E Light Sch of PN Metro Sch Dist Mrs Karen Selwa Williams, Dir *Chair's #: (317) 259-5265 Ext 4017*	1901 E 86 St Indianapolis	46240				TCH	PBL			Publication withheld			
004	Marion Comm Sch-Tuckr Area V-T Ctr Mrs Joyce Dolby, Dir *Chair's #: (765) 664-9091*	107 S Pennsylvania Ave Marion	46952				TCH	PBL	12	12	31	32	26	32
029	St Anthony Medical Center Ms Carol Anderson, Director *Chair's #: (219) 757-6480*	203 Franciscan Dr Crown Point	46307				HSP	PVT			Publication withheld			
015	Vincennes Univ, Practical Nsg Program Ms Karen R Gines, Chair *Chair's #: (812) 888-4325*	1002 North First St Vincennes	47591			A	CC	PBL	11	12	24	31	20	25
021	Vincennes Univ-Jasper Campus Mrs Mary Price, Chair *Chair's #: (812) 481-5926*	850 College Ave Jasper	47546				CC	PBL	13	12	17	18	15	18

Explanation of footnotes on page x

School Code	Name of School, Director of Program, and Phone Number	Street Address / City or Town and Zip Code	Footnotes	Type of Program	NLNAC Accreditation as of January 31, 1999	Administrative Control	Financial Support (principal source)	Number of Months in Program	Educational Requirements for Entering Adult Program	Enrollments as of October 15, 1998	Admissions Aug. 1, 1997 - July 31, 1998	Graduations Aug. 1, 1997 - July 31, 1998	Fall Admissions Aug. 1, 1998 - Dec. 31, 1998
	IOWA												
	29 Programs in 29 Schools												
012	Des Moines Area Comm Coll-Boone Ms Susan Wager, Director *Chair's #: (515) 964-6316*	1125 Hancock Dr Boone 50036			A	CC	PBL	9	12	36	35	36	1
006	Des Moines Area Comm College-Anken Ms Susan Wager, Director *Chair's #: (515) 964-6316*	2006 S Ankeny Blvd 9 Ankeny 50021			A	CC	PBL	9	12	71	71	60	0
007	Des Moines Area Comm College-Carroll Ms Susan Wager, Director *Chair's #: (515) 964-6316*	906 N Grant Rd Carroll 51401			A	CC	PBL	9	12	15	23	22	0
026	Des Moines Central Campus Mrs Martha A Schaer, Coord *Chair's #: (515) 242-7846 Ext 3462*	1800 Grand Ave Des Moines 50309	HS			SEC SEC	PBL PBL	18		0 14	0 4	0 9	0 12
009	Eastern Iowa CC Dist-Clinton CC Ms Nancy E Knutstrom, Coord *Chair's #: (319) 244 Ext 384*	1000 Lincoln Blvd Clinton 52732				CC	PBL			Publication withheld			
008	Eastern Iowa CC Dist-Scott CC Ms Nancy E Knutstrom, Coord *Chair's #: (319) 359-7531 Ext 304*	500 Belmont Rd Bettendorf 52722				CC	PBL			Publication withheld			
005	Hawkeye Comm College Mrs Brenda Hempen, Coord *Chair's #: (319) 296-4013 Ext 1469*	1501 E Orange Rd Box 8015 Waterloo 50704				CC	PBL	12	12	196	100	65	60
010	Indian Hills CC-Ottumwa Ms M Ann Aulwes, Chair *Chair's #: (515) 683-5165 Ext 5165*	525 Grandview Ottumwa 52501				CC	PBL			Publication withheld			
014	Indian Hills Comm College-Centerville Ms M Ann Aulwes, Chair *Chair's #: (515) 683-5111 Ext 5165*	721 N First St Centerville 52544				CC	PBL			Publication withheld			
031	Iowa Central CC-Webster City Mrs Diane Sorensen, Coord *Chair's #: (515) 832-1632*	1725 Beach St Webster City 50595	7			CC	PBL			Data reported w/AD prog			
028	Iowa Central Comm College Mrs Brenda Gleason, Dir *Chair's #: (515) 576-7201 Ext 2310*	916 N Russell St Storm Lake 50588	7			CC	PBL			Data reported w/AD prog			
021	Iowa Central Comm College-Fort Dodge Mrs Brenda Gleason, Dir *Chair's #: (515) 576-0099 Ext 2310*	330 Ave M Fort Dodge 50501				CC	PBL	10	12	15	11	25	1
015	Iowa Lakes Comm College Mrs Judi Donahue, Dir *Chair's #: (712) 852-5285*	3200 College Dr Emmetsburg 50536				CC	PBL	10	12	54	46	40	56

Explanation of footnotes on page x

School Code	Name of School, Director of Program, and Phone Number	Street Address City or Town and Zip Code	Footnotes	Type of Program	NLNAC Accreditation as of January 31, 1999	Administrative Control	Financial Support (principal source)	Number of Months in Program	Educational Requirements for Entering Adult Program	Enrollments as of October 15, 1998	Admissions Aug. 1, 1997 - July 31, 1998	Graduations Aug. 1, 1997 - July 31, 1998	Fall Admissions Aug. 1, 1998 - Dec. 31, 1998
	IOWA												
	- Continued												
001	Iowa Valley Comm College (2 Campuse Mrs Mavis A Hunt, Coord *Chair's #: (515) 752-7106 Ext 297*	3700 S Center St Marshalltown 50158				CC	PBL			Publication withheld			
019	Iowa Western Comm Coll Council Bluff Ms Carol Maxwell, Coord *Chair's #: (712) 325-3200 Ext 352*	2700 College Rd Box 4-C Council Bluffs 51502	7			TCH	PBL			Data reported w/AD prog			
004	Iowa Western Comm College-Clarinda Ms Roberta Kokenge, Coord *Chair's #: (712) 542-5117 Ext 0240*	923 E Washington Clarinda 51632				TCH	PBL	11	12	31	36	30	0
027	Iowa Western Comm College-Harlan Ms Sue Smith, Coord *Chair's #: (712) 755-3568*	2712 12th St Harlan 51537				CC	PBL	11	12	10	13	11	10
017	Kirkwood Comm College Ms Linda Schwartz, Coord *Chair's #: (319) 398-5630*	6301 Kirkwood Blvd SW Bx 20 Cedar Rapids 52406	7			CC	PBL			Data reported w/AD prog			
011	North Iowa Area Comm College Mrs Donna J Orton, Chair *Chair's #: (515) 422-4216*	500 College Dr Mason City 50401				CC	PBL	10	12	22	18	16	23
023	Northeast Iowa Comm Coll-Calmar Mrs Melinda Hanson, Chair *Chair's #: (319) 562-3263 Ext 262*	Box 400 Hwy 150 South Calmar 52132	7	HSE		CC CC	PBL PBL			Datareported w/ADprog			
020	Northeast Iowa Comm Coll-Peosta Mrs Geraldine Althoff, Dir *Chair's #: (319) 556-5110 Ext 209*	10250 Sundown Rd Peosta 52068				CC	PBL			Publication withheld			
030	Northwest Iowa Comm College Mrs Mary C Mohni, Dir *Chair's #: (712) 324-5061 Ext 117*	Hwy 18 West Sheldon 51201				CC	PBL	11	12	32	39	31	39
016	Southeastern Comm College-Burlington Ms Pamela Bradley, Dir *Chair's #: (319) 752-2731 Ext 8164*	1015 S Gear Ave West Burlington 52655				CC	PBL			28	13	9	0
029	Southeastern Comm College-Keokuk Dr. Lee Alderman, Dean *Chair's #: (800) 828-7322 Ext 8277*	335 Messenger Rd Box 6007 Keokuk 52632	7			CC	PBL			Data reported w/AD prog			
024	Southwestern Comm College Mrs Loretta A Eckels, Chair *Chair's #: (515) 782-7081 Ext 271*	1501 W Townline Rd Creston 50801				CC	PBL			Publication withheld			
013	Western Iowa Tech CC (2 Campuses) Mrs. Barbara A Condon, Chair *Chair's #: (712) 274-8733 Ext 1356*	4647 Stone Ave Box 265 Sioux City 51102			A	CC	PBL	9	12	121	115	98	79

Explanation of footnotes on page x

KANSAS

19 Programs in 18 Schools

School Code	Name of School, Director of Program, and Phone Number	Street Address / City or Town and Zip Code	Footnotes	Type of Program	NLNAC Accreditation as of January 31, 1999	Administrative Control	Financial Support (principal source)	Number of Months in Program	Educational Requirements for Entering Adult Program	Enrollments as of October 15, 1998	Admissions Aug. 1, 1997 - July 31, 1998	Graduations Aug. 1, 1997 - July 31, 1998	Fall Admissions Aug. 1, 1998 - Dec. 31, 1998
020	Barton Co Comm College / Ms Karla Homan, Director / Chair's #: (316) 792-9355	Great Bend 67530				CC	PBL	12	12	27	26	24	36
021	Butler Co Comm College / Ms Patricia Bayles, Dean / Chair's #: (316) 322-3146	901 S Haverhill Rd / El Dorado 67042	7			CC	PBL			Data reported w/AD prog			
012	Colby Community College / Mrs Janet Myers, Dir / Chair's #: (785) 462-3984 Ext 319	1255 S Range / Colby 67701			A	CC	PBL			Data reported w/AD prog			
005	Dodge City Community College / Mrs Linda K Sanko, Director / Chair's #: (316) 225-1321 Ext 226	2501 N 14th Ave / Dodge City 67801			A	CC	PBL	10	12	37	38 —	34	37
008	Flint Hills Tech Coll / Mrs Kathleen Bode, Chair / Chair's #: (316) 341-2300 Ext 226	3301 W 18th / Emporia 66801				TCH	PBL	11	12	35	43	34	24
027	Hutchinson Comm Coll / Mrs Brenda L Moffitt, Dir / Chair's #: (316) 241-4417	925 N Walnut / McPherson 67460			A	CC	PBL	10	12	32	30	24	34
007	Johnson County Comm College/AVS / Dr Ann Hess, Coord / Chair's #: (913) 649-2383	10000 W 75 N St Suite 241 / Merriam 66204				CC	PBL	10	12	19	21	17	24
016	Kansas City, KS Area Voc-Tech Sch / Ms Susan White, Supv / Chair's #: (913) 596-5500 Ext 332	2220 N 59th St / Kansas City 66104				TCH	PBL	11	12	72	94	59	53
004	KAW Area Tech School-Dept of PN / Dr Julie Putnam, Coord / Chair's #: (785) 228-6308	5724 Huntoon / Topeka 66604	HSE		A / A	TCH / TCH	PBL / PBL	10 / 10	12 / 12	60 / 1	76 / 2	46 / 0	32 / 0
022	Labette Comm College / Ms Patricia Thompson, Dir / Chair's #: (316) 421-6700 Ext 62	200 South 14th St / Parsons 67357				CC	PBL			43	45	34	43
011	Manhattan Area Tech Coll / Mrs Myrna J Bartel, Coord / Chair's #: (785) 587-2800 Ext 121	3136 Dickens / Manhattan 66503				TCH	PBL	11	12	44	44	42	45
006	Neosho County Comm Jr College / Ms Carol Fox, Dir / Chair's #: (316) 431-2820 Ext 255	800 West 14th / Chanute 66720	7			CC	PBL			Data reported with/AD pro			
013	No Ctrl KS Cloud Co Comm Coll / Mrs Vera Streit, Coord / Chair's #: (785) 738-9025	Box 507 / Beloit 67420			A	TCH	PBL	11	12	39	28	23	40

Explanation of footnotes on page x

School Code	Name of School, Director of Program, and Phone Number	Street Address, City or Town and Zip Code	Footnotes	Type of Program	NLNAC Accreditation as of January 31, 1999	Administrative Control	Financial Support (principal source)	Number of Months in Program	Educational Requirements for Entering Adult Program	Enrollments as of October 15, 1998	Admissions Aug. 1, 1997 - July 31, 1998	Graduations Aug. 1, 1997 - July 31, 1998	Fall Admissions Aug. 1, 1998 - Dec. 31, 1998
	KANSAS												
	- Continued												
001	North Central Ks Area Tech College Ms Sandra Gottschalk, Dir *Chair's #: (785) 623-6175*	2205 Wheatlamd Ave Hays 69601				TCH	PBL			Publication withheld			
014	Northeast Kansas Area Tech Sch Ms Janean Bowen, Supv *Chair's #: (913) 367-6204 Ext 134*	1501 W Riley Atchison 66002				TCH	PBL	11	12	26	30	21	0
023	Pratt Comm College Mrs Diane Okeson, Dean *Chair's #: (316) 672-5641 Ext 232*	348 NE State Rd 61 Pratt 67124	7			CC	PBL			Data reported w/AD prog			
019	Seward County Community College Mr Steve Hecox, Chair *Chair's #: (316) 626-3026*	Box 1137 Liberal 67901				CC	PBL	10	12	24	25	24	25
003	Wichita Area Tech College Mrs Donna Granger, Specialist *Chair's #: (316) 833-4374*	324 N Emporia Wichita 67202			A	TCH	PBL	11	12	60	64	52	43
	KENTUCKY												
	24 Programs in 18 Schools												
021	Ashland Tech College Ms Vicki Hemlepp, Coord *Chair's #: (606) 928-6427 Ext 261*	4818 Roberts Dr Ashland 41102				TCH	PBL	15	12	30	40	18	0
009	Bowling Green Tech Coll-Glasgow Mrs Rebecca S Forrest, Director *Chair's #: (502) 651-5673*	129 State Ave Glasgow 42141				TCH	PBL	15	12	32	59	46	33
007	Cental KY Tech Coll--Danville Mrs Sandra Houston, Director *Chair's #: (606) 239-7030*	1714 Perryville Rd Danville 40423				TCH	PBL	12	12	95	134	39	37
004	Central KY Tech College Ms Bonnie Nicholson, Chair *Chair's #: (606) 246-2400*	308 Voc Tech Rd Lexington 40511				TCH	PBL			49	74	35	27
016	Cumberland Vly Tech College Mrs Margaret Peace, Admin *Chair's #: (606) 337-3106 Ext 0020*	US 25E Box 187 Pineville 40977				TCH	PBL	11	12	82	66	24	43
001	Elizabethtown Tech Coll Mrs Maurita Roper, Coord *Chair's #: (502) 766-5133 Ext 119*	505 University Dr Elizabethtown 42701				TCH	PBL	18	12	23	21	19	23
019	Hazard Tech College Mrs Phyllis Morris, Dept Chair *Chair's #: (606) 435-6101 Ext 166*	101 Vo-Tech Drive Hazard 41701				TCH	PBL	18	12	71	70	47	24

School Code	Name of School, Director of Program, and Phone Number	Street Address / City or Town and Zip Code	Footnotes	Type of Program	NLNAC Accreditation as of January 31, 1999	Administrative Control	Financial Support (principal source)	Number of Months in Program	Educational Requirements for Entering Adult Program	Enrollments as of October 15, 1998	Admissions Aug. 1, 1997 - July 31, 1998	Graduations Aug. 1, 1997 - July 31, 1998	Fall Admissions Aug. 1, 1998 - Dec. 31, 1998
	KENTUCKY												
	- Continued												
010	Jefferson Tech College Mrs Jane A Hudson, Coord *Chair's #: (502) 595-4275*	800 W Chestnut St Louisville 40203	HS			TCH TCH	PBL PBL	15	12 12	36 7	64 8	35 6	28 8
022	Kentucky Tech -Murray Ms Rhanda Miller, Coord *Chair's #: (502) 753-1870*	18th & Sycamore Murray 42071				TCH	PBL			Publication withheld			
020	Madisonville Tech Coll Mrs Elaine Terry, Coord *Chair's #: (502) 824-7552 Ext 183*	750 N Laffoon St Madisonville 42431				TCH	PBL	13	12	35	53	27	21
006	Mayo Tech Coll Ms Sue Garland, Dept Chair *Chair's #: (606) 789-5321 Ext 246*	W 3rd St Paintsville 41240				TCH	PBL	15		45	40	25	31
018	Norther KY Tech Coll Ms Georgianne Duffy, Coord *Chair's #: (606) 341-5200*	790 Thomas More Parkway Edgewood 41017				TCH	PBL			50	31	30	27
015	Owensboro Tech Coll Ms Nancy Turner, Chair *Chair's #: (502) 687-7322 Ext 147*	1501 Frederica St Owensboro 42301				TCH	PBL	9		27	20	19	30
053	Rowan Tech College Mrs Claudia Collins, Coord *Chair's #: (606) 783-1538 Ext 305*	609 Viking Dr Morehead 40351				TCH	PBL	15	12	36	55	30	0
051	Somerset Tech College Ms Ruth Martin, Coord *Chair's #: (606) 677-4049 Ext 126*	230 Airport Rd Somerset 42501				TCH	PBL	0	12	72	36	55	36
049	Spencerian College Mrs L Newton, Dir *Chair's #: (502) 447-1000 Ext 213*	4627 Dixie Highway Louisville 40216				IND	PVT	12	12	130	151	118	30
900	The Health Inst of Louisville Ms Patricia Recktenwald, Dir *Chair's #: (502) 580-3660*	612 S Fourth Ave Louisville 40202				TCH	PVT			89	141	83	64
023	West KY Tech Coll Mrs Marie Thieleman, Coord *Chair's #: (502) 554-6270*	5200 Blandville Rd PO Box 74 Paducah 42002				TCH	PBL	9	12	22	17	9	23
	LOUISIANA												
	48 Programs in 46 Schools												
065	Cameron College Dr Lynn Tarzetti, Dir *Chair's #: (504) 821-5881*	2740 Canal St New Orleans 70119				CC	PVT			Publication withheld			

School Code	Name of School, Director of Program, and Phone Number	Street Address / City or Town and Zip Code		Footnotes	Type of Program	NLNAC Accreditation as of January 31, 1999	Administrative Control	Financial Support (principal source)	Number of Months in Program	Educational Requirements for Entering Adult Program	Enrollments as of October 15, 1998	Admissions Aug. 1, 1997 - July 31, 1998	Graduations Aug. 1, 1997 - July 31, 1998	Fall Admissions Aug. 1, 1998 - Dec. 31, 1998
	LOUISIANA													
	- Continued													
052	Delgado Comm Coll Mrs Gayle Barrau, Dean Chair's #: (504) 483-4666 Ext 4646	980 Navarre Ave New Orleans	70124				TCH	PBL			38	53	37	10
082	Delta College of Arts and Technology Ms Debra Courtade, Coord Chair's #: (225) 927-7780 Ext 14	7290 Exchange Pl Baton Rouge	70806				TCH	PVT			Publication withheld			
047	Elaine P Nunez Comm College Ms Andrea Phillipi, Coord Chair's #: (504) 278-7440	3700 La Fontaine St Chalmette	70043				TCH	PBL			Publication withheld			
068	LA Tech Coll -Mansfield Campus Ms Camillia Spilker, Dept Head Chair's #: (318) 872-2243	PO Box 1236 Mansfield	71052				TCH	PBL			Publication withheld			
007	LA Tech Coll-Delta-Ouachita Campus Mrs Paula Ott Nisbet, Dept Head Chair's #: (318) 397-6100 Ext 221	609 Vocational Pky West Monroe	71291				TCH	PBL			140	214	78	64
055	LA Tech Coll-Evangeline Campus Mrs Etta Ramona Hamilton, Coord Chair's #: (318) 394-6466 Ext 19	PO Box 68 St Martinville	70582				TCH	PBL			Publication withheld			
046	LA Tech Coll-Florida Pariches Mr George Foster, Dir Chair's #: (225) 222-4351	PO Box 130 Greensburg	70441				TCH	PBL			Publication withheld			
043	LA Tech Coll-Folkes Campus Mrs Faith Rohner, Dir Chair's #: (225) 634-2636	PO Box 808 Jackson	70748				TCH	PBL			Publication withheld			
022	LA Tech Coll-Gulf Area Campus Mrs Amy M Sellers, Dept Head Chair's #: (318) 893-4984	PO Box 878 Abbeville	70510				TCH	PBL			31	51	18	0
020	LA Tech Coll-Hammond Area Campus Mrs Roberta Connelley, Coord Chair's #: (504) 543-4120	PO Box 489 Hammond	70404				TCH	PBL			Publication withheld			
036	LA Tech Coll-Huey P Long Campus Mrs Evelyn Hyde, Coord Chair's #: (318) 628-4342	303 S Jones St Winnfield	71483				TCH	PBL			Publication withheld			
018	LA Tech Coll-Jefferson Campus Mrs Sandra Dawes, Coord Chair's #: (504) 736-7086	5200 Blair Dr Metairie	70001				TCH	PBL			76	91	70	0
056	LA Tech Coll-Jefferson Davis Campus Mr Johnnie Smith, Dir Chair's #: (318) 824-4811	1230 N Main St PO Box 1327 Jenning	70546				TCH	PBL			Publication withheld			

Explanation of footnotes on page x

LOUISIANA

- Continued

School Code	Name of School, Director of Program, and Phone Number	Street Address / City or Town and Zip Code		Footnotes	Type of Program	NLNAC Accreditation as of January 31, 1999	Administrative Control	Financial Support (principal source)	Number of Months in Program	Educational Requirements for Entering Adult Program	Enrollments as of October 15, 1998	Admissions Aug. 1, 1997 - July 31, 1998	Graduations Aug. 1, 1997 - July 31, 1998	Fall Admissions Aug. 1, 1998 - Dec. 31, 1998
050	LA Tech Coll-Lafayette Campus Mrs Pemella Williams, Dept Head *Chair's #: (318) 262-5962*	PO Box 4909 Lafayette	70502				TCH	PBL			Publication withheld			
062	LA Tech Coll-Lafourche Campus Mrs Myra Cheramie, Dept Head *Chair's #: (504) 447-0924*	1425 Tiger Dr Box 1831 Thibodaux	70302				TCH	PBL	14	12	17	22	17	17
045	LA Tech Coll-Lamar Salter Campus Ms Patricia Nunnally, Coord *Chair's #: (318) 537-3135*	15014 Lake Charles Hwy Leesville	71446				TCH	PBL	14	12	17	39	22	0
024	LA Tech Coll-Natchitoches Campus Mrs Melanie McMillin, Coord *Chair's #: (318) 357-3162*	PO Box 657 Natchitoches	71457				TCH	PBL			25	37	0	0
035	LA Tech Coll-Northeast LA Campus Mrs Beverly Peoples, Coord *Chair's #: (318) 435-2163*	1710 Warren St Winnsboro	71295				TCH	PBL	18	12	21	0	15	27
044	LA Tech Coll-Northwest LA Campus Mrs Sharon Turley, Dept Head *Chair's #: (318) 927-3035*	PO Box 835 Minden	71058				TCH	PBL			Publication withheld			
058	LA Tech Coll-Oakdale Campus Mrs Rebecca Harrell, Dept Head *Chair's #: (318) 335-3944*	PO Drawer E M Oakdale	71463				TCH	PBL			Publication withheld			
042	LA Tech Coll-Ruston Campus Mrs Janet Armstrong, Coordinator *Chair's #: (318) 251-4145*	PO Box 1070 Ruston	71273				TCH	PBL	16	12	15	29	22	0
001	LA Tech Coll-Shreveport-Bossier Camp Mrs Ann Caskey Ryals, Coord *Chair's #: (318) 676-7811*	2010 N Market St Shreveport	71107				TCH	PBL			Publication withheld			
028	LA Tech Coll-Sidney N Collins Campus Mrs Desaree Holmes, Dept Head *Chair's #: (504) 942-8333*	3727 Louisa St New Orleans	70126				TCH	PBL			Publication withheld			
034	LA Tech Coll-Slidell Campus Mrs Barbara Holloway, Dept Head *Chair's #: (504) 646-6430*	PO Box 827 Slidell	70459				TCH	PBL	18	12	26	43	15	0
025	LA Tech Coll-South LA Campus Mrs Donna Leach Kane, Dept Head *Chair's #: (504) 857-3655*	PO Box 5033 Houma	70361				TCH	PBL	15	12	26	37	28	31
006	LA Tech Coll-Sowela Campus Mrs Phyllis Robinson, Dept Head *Chair's #: (318) 491-2696*	3820 Legion St Lake Charles	70601				TCH	PBL			58	90	58	45

Explanation of footnotes on page x

School Code	Name of School, Director of Program, and Phone Number	Street Address City or Town and Zip Code		Footnotes	Type of Program	NLNAC Accreditation as of January 31, 1999	Administrative Control	Financial Support (principal source)	Number of Months in Program	Educational Requirements for Entering Adult Program	Enrollments as of October 15, 1998	Admissions Aug. 1, 1997 - July 31, 1998	Graduations Aug. 1, 1997 - July 31, 1998	Fall Admissions Aug. 1, 1998 - Dec. 31, 1998
	LOUISIANA													
	- Continued													
015	LA Tech Coll-Sullivan Campus Ms Judy Wamsley, Dept Head *Chair's #: (504) 732-6640 Ext 23*	1710 Sullivan Dr Bogalusa	70427				TCH	PBL			Publication withheld			
012	LA Tech Coll-T H Harris Campus Mrs Laurie Fontenot, Dept Head *Chair's #: (318) 948-0336*	337 E South St Opelousas	70570				TCH	PBL			Publication withheld			
049	LA Tech Coll-Tallulah Campus Mrs Margaret Shoemaker, Coord *Chair's #: (318) 574-4820 Ext 0007*	PO Drawer 1740 Tallulah	71282				TCH	PBL			Publication withheld			
038	LA Tech Coll-W Jefferson Campus Ms Ruth Finney, Head *Chair's #: (504) 361-6471*	475 Manhattan Blvd Harvey	70058				TCH	PBL			Publication withheld			
026	LA Tech Coll-Westside Campus Mr Alfred Bell, Dir *Chair's #: (225) 687-6392*	PO Box 733 Plaquemine	70764				TCH	PBL			Publication withheld			
021	LA Tech Coll-Young Memorial Campus Mr Gregory Garrett, Dir *Chair's #: (504) 380-2436*	PO Box 2148 Morgan City	70380				TCH	PBL			Publication withheld			
066	LA Tech College At Ville Platte Mr Mark A Doucet, Coord *Chair's #: (318) 363-2197 Ext 135*	PO Box 296 Ville Platte	70586				TCH	PBL			Publication withheld			
014	LA Tech College-Alexandria Campus Ms Stephanie Jackson, Dept Head *Chair's #: (318) 487-5435*	4311 S MacArthur Dr Alexandria	71301				TCH	PBL			Publication withheld			
051	LA Tech College-Avoyelles Campus Mrs Kate Moreau, Coord *Chair's #: (318) 563-8685*	PO Box 307 Cottonport	73127				TCH	PBL			Publication withheld			
008	LA Tech College-Baton Rouge Campus Ms Beverly W McNeese, Dept Head *Chair's #: (225) 359-9201*	3250 N Acadian Hwy Baton Rouge	70805				TCH	PBL			Publication withheld			
900	LA Tech College-Clairborne Campus Ms Melinda Parnell, Coord *Chair's #: (318) 927-2034*	3001 Minden Rd Homer	71050				TCH	PBL			Publication withheld			
004	LA Technical Coll-S Jackson Campus Mrs Mignonne Ater, Coord *Chair's #: (318) 757-6501*	Po Box 152 Ferriday	71334				TCH	PBL			Publication withheld			
019	LA Technical Coll-Teche Area Campus Ms Vickie Migues, Coord *Chair's #: (318) 373-0011*	PO Box 1057 New Iberia	70562				TCH	PBL			29	86	31	46

Explanation of footnotes on page x

School Code	Name of School, Director of Program, and Phone Number	Street Address / City or Town and Zip Code		Footnotes	Type of Program	NLNAC Accreditation as of January 31, 1999	Administrative Control	Financial Support (principal source)	Number of Months in Program	Educational Requirements for Entering Adult Program	Enrollments as of October 15, 1998	Admissions Aug. 1, 1997 - July 31, 1998	Graduations Aug. 1, 1997 - July 31, 1998	Fall Admissions Aug. 1, 1998 - Dec. 31, 1998
	LOUISIANA													
	- Continued													
040	LA Technical College Bastrop Ms Tammy Le Bleu, Instructor *Chair's #: (318) 283-0836 Ext 21*	PO Box 1120 Bastrop	71220				TCH	PBL			38	44	26	38
063	LA Technical College-North Central Mrs Carolyn Yakaboski, Dir *Chair's #: (318) 368-3179*	PO Box 548 Farmerville	71241				TCH	PBL	15	12	16	30	15	32
016	LA Technical College-Reserve Mrs Jean Houin, Coord *Chair's #: (504) 536-4418 Ext 216*	181 Regala Pk Reserve	70084				TCH	PBL			10	30	12	0
005	LA-Tech College-Acadian Campus Mrs Rosalyn Z Baty, Dept Head *Chair's #: (318) 788-7521*	1933 W Hutchinson Ave Crowley	70526				TCH	PVT			Publication withheld			
009	Lafayette Gen Med Center Mrs Heidi H Benoit, Coord *Chair's #: (318) 289-8980*	1214 Coolidge Lafayette	70505				HSP	PBL	13	12	23	38	22	38
048	LTC, Jumonville-Memorial Campus Mr Tommy Gauthier, Dir *Chair's #: (504) 638-8613 Ext 12*	PO Box 725 New Roads	70760				TCH	PBL			Publication withheld			
	MAINE													
	5 Programs in 5 Schools													
005	Central Maine Tech College Ms Anne Schuettinger, Chair *Chair's #: (207) 755-5408*	1250 Turner St Auburn	04210		7			CC	PBL			Data reported w/AD Prog			
006	Eastern Maine Tech College Ms Marilyn A Lavelle, Chair *Chair's #: (207) 941-4600 Ext 4657*	354 Hogan Rd Bangor	04401		7			TCH	PBL			Data reported w/AD prog			
002	Kennebec Valley Tech College Mrs Marcia Parker, Chair *Chair's #: (207) 453-5167*	92 Western Ave Fairfield	04937		7			TCH	PBL			Data reported w/AD Prog			
001	Northern Maine Tech College Mrs B Kent Conant, Chair *Chair's #: (207) 768-2749*	33 Edgemont Dr Presque Isle	04769		7			TCH	PBL			Data reported w/AD Prog			
003	Southern Maine Tech College Mrs Nancy Smith, Chair *Chair's #: (207) 767-9588*	Fort Rd South Portland	04106		7			CC	PBL			Data reported w/AD prog			
	MARYLAND													
	13 Programs in 13 Schools													
043	Allegany Coll of Maryland Mrs Fran Leibfreid, Dir *Chair's #: (301) 784-5568*	12401 Willowbrook Rd Cumberland	21502		7			CC	PBL			Data reported w/AD prog			

School Code	Name of School, Director of Program, and Phone Number	Street Address / City or Town and Zip Code	Footnotes	Type of Program	NLNAC Accreditation as of January 3, 1999	Administrative Control	Financial Support (principal source)	Number of Months in Program	Educational Requirements for Entering Adult Program	Enrollments as of October 15, 1998	Admissions Aug. 1, 1997 - July 31, 1998	Graduations Aug. 1, 1997 - July 31, 1998	Fall Admissions Aug. 1, 1998 - Dec. 31, 1998
	MARYLAND **- Continued**												
002	Baltimore City Comm Coll Ms Dorothy Holley, Chair *Chair's #: (410) 462-7765*	2901 Liberty Hts Ave Baltimore 21215	1			CC	PBL			Publication withheld			
017	Baltimore City Public Sch-PN Ms Barbara Kinder, Nurse Admin *Chair's #: (410) 396-7267*	4501 Edmoson Ave Baltimore 21229				SEC	PBL			Publication withheld			
036	Carroll County Career & Tech Center Mrs Catherine Engel, Principal *Chair's #: (410) 751-3669*	Westminster 21157		HS		SEC SEC	PBL PBL	120		0 17	0 22	0 7	0 19
050	Cecil Comm College Mrs Mary Way Bolt, Dir *Chair's #: (410) 287-6060 Ext 333*	1000 North East Rd North East 21901	7			CC	PBL			Data reported w/AD prog			
042	Charles County Community College Ms Margaret DeStefanis, Chair *Chair's #: (301) 934-7535*	Mitchell Rd, Box 910 La Plata 20646			A	CC	PBL	11	12	10	20	18	11
001	Chesapeake College Dr Maurice Hickey, Assoc Dean *Chair's #: (410) 827-5927*	PO Box 8 Wye Mills 21676	1			CC	PBL			Publication withheld			
048	Fredreick Comm Coll PN prog Ms Jane Garvin, Dir *Chair's #: (301) 846-2525*	7932 Opossumtown Pike Fredrick 21702	7			CC	PBL			Data reported w/AD prog			
044	Harford Comm College PN Prog Ms Joyce Jordon, Chair *Chair's #: (410) 836-4389*	401 Thomas Run Rd Bel Air 21014	7			CC	PBL			Data reported w/AD prog			
051	Howard Comm Coll Dr Emily Slunt, Chair *Chair's #: (410) 772-4888*	Little Patuyent Pkwy Columbia 21044			A	CC	PBL	11	12	24	17	24	17
040	PN Program Center for Applied Tech Mrs Mary Campbell, Chair *Chair's #: (969) 969-3100 Ext 206*	Stevenson Rd-Rt 7-Bx 265 Severn 21144		HS HSE		TCH TCH TCH	PBL PBL PBL	18	10 10	5 40	4 26	5 17	2 23
052	Prince George's Comm Coll Dr Lois Neuman, Chair *Chair's #: (301) 322-0734*	301 Largo Rd Largo 20774	7			CC	PBL			Data reported w/AD prog			
045	Wor-Wic Comm College Nsg Dept Ms Denise Marshall, Dept Head *Chair's #: (410) 221-2555*	Eshc-PO Box 800 Cambridge 21613				CC	PBL			Publication withheld			

Explanation of footnotes on page x

MASSACHUSETTS

27 Programs in 21 Schools

School Code	Name of School, Director of Program, and Phone Number	Street Address / City or Town and Zip Code		Footnotes	Type of Program	NLNAC Accreditation as of January 31, 1999	Administrative Control	Financial Support (principal source)	Number of Months in Program	Educational Requirements for Entering Adult Program	Enrollments as of October 15, 1998	Admissions Aug. 1, 1997 - July 31, 1998	Graduations Aug. 1, 1997 - July 31, 1998	Fall Admissions Aug. 1, 1998 - Dec. 31, 1998
050	Assabet Valley Reg Voc Sch Mrs Joan Kilroy, Coord Chair's #: (508) 485-9430 Ext 0471	Fitchburg St Marlboro	01752				TCH	PBL	10	12	35	40	28	45
055	Berkshire Comm College Dr Margaret Chalmers, Chair Chair's #: (413) 499-4660 Ext 450	343 Main St Great Barrington	01230				CC	PBL	10	12	17	24	13	21
027	Blue Hills Regional Tech Sch Mrs Maureen McCann, Chair Chair's #: (617) 828-5800 Ext 305	800 Randolph St Canton	02021				TCH	PVT			39	30	33	39
049	Bristol-Plymouth Reg Voc-Tech Sch Mrs Carolyn Pearson, Dir Chair's #: (508) 823-5151 Ext 240	940 County St Taunton	02780				TCH	PBL	10	12	40	40	34	42
026	Diman Reg Voc-Tech Sch Ms Barbara Pitera, Director Chair's #: (508) 678-2891 Ext 156	251Stonehaven Rd Fall River	02723				TCH	PVT	10	12	46	49	40	49
029	EATI PN Prog Mrs Donna Lampman, Dept Head Chair's #: (978) 774-0050 Ext 270	562 Maple St Hathorne	01937				TCH	PBL			Publication withheld			
053	Greater Lowell Reg Voc-Tech Sch Ms Nancy Harrington, Dir Chair's #: (978) 441-0990 Ext 225	Pawtucket Blvd Tyngsboro	01879				TCH	PVT	10	12	78	80	69	80
028	Greenfield Comm College-PN Prog Ms Virginia Wahl, Coord Chair's #: (413) 586-9771	80 Locust St Northampton	01060				CC	PBL	10	12	31	29	24	31
019	Lemuel Shattuck Hosp Sch of PN Dr Mary Keaveny, Dir Chair's #: (617) 522-8110 Ext 244	180 Morton St Jamaica Plain	02130				HSP	PBL			Publication withheld			
056	MA Bay Comm College Ms Elleen Andrews O'Brien, Chair Chair's #: (508) 270-4257	19 Flagg Drive Framingham	01701				CC	PBL	10	12	78	82	54	87
002	Montachusett RVTS Ms Marjorie Tremblay, Director Chair's #: (978) 345-9200 Ext 107	1050 Westmister St Fitchburg	01420	1			TCH	PBL	10	12	26	27	0	27
054	Northern Essex Comm College Mrs Flora S McLaughlin, Chair Chair's #: (978) 738-7446	Elliot Way Haverhill	01830			A	CC	PBL	10	12	45	38	26	45
041	Quincy College Mrs Marybeth Pepin, Chair Chair's #: (617) 984-1692	34 Coddington St Quincy	02169			A	CC	PBL			118	90	78	120

School Code	Name of School, Director of Program, and Phone Number	Street Address / City or Town and Zip Code		Footnotes	Type of Program	NLNAC Accreditation as of January 31, 1999	Administrative Control	Financial Support (principal source)	Number of Months in Program	Educational Requirements for Entering Adult Program	Enrollments as of October 15, 1998	Admissions Aug. 1, 1997 - July 31, 1998	Graduations Aug. 1, 1997 - July 31, 1998	Fall Admissions Aug. 1, 1998 - Dec. 31, 1998
	MASSACHUSETTS													
	- Continued													
001	Shawsheen Valley T H S Mrs Barbara Ahern, Coord *Chair's #: (978) 663-2722*	100 Cook St Billerica	01821					TCH	PBL	10	12	42	42	36	42
020	Soldiers' Home Mrs Kathleen Arinello, Dir *Chair's #: (617) 884-5660 Ext 627*	91 Crest Ave Chelsea	02150				A	HSP	PBL	10	12	30	40	32	34
034	Southeastern Reg Voc-Tech Sch Mrs Hilary Hamilton, Director *Chair's #: (508) 230-9241*	250 Foundry St South Easton	02375					TCH	PBL	10	12	38	68	52	38
044	Upper Cape Cod Reg Tech Sch Dr Joan Bruce, Coordinator *Chair's #: (508) 759-7711 Ext 285*	220 Sandwich Rd Bourne	02532					TCH	PBL			Publication withheld			
037	William J Dean Tech HS Miss Eleanor A Hepburn, Director *Chair's #: (413) 534-2086*	1045 Main St Holyoke	01040					TCH	PBL	10	12	30	30	28	30
018	Worcester Tech Inst Mrs Junea M Hutchins, Dept Head *Chair's #: (508) 799-1947*	251 Belmont St Worcester	01605					TCH	PBL			Publication withheld			
007	Youville Hosp Sch of Practical Nursing Ms Helen M Barrett, Director *Chair's #: (617) 964-4144*	15 Walnut Park Newton	02158				A	HSP	PVT	10	12	25	52	14	0
	MICHIGAN													
	27 Programs in 27 Schools													
042	Alpena Comm College Mrs Kathleen McGillis, Asst Dean *Chair's #: (517) 356-9021 Ext 226*	666 Johnson St Alpena	49707	7			CC	PBL	10	12	34	28	27	36	
033	Bay de Noc Comm College Mrs Patricia Valensky, Dean *Chair's #: (800) 221-2001 Ext 1208*	2001 North Lincoln Rd Escanaba	49829				CC	PBL	12	12	100	52	57	61	
014	Bay Mills Comm Coll Ms Terri Waisanew, Dir *Chair's #: (906) 248-5843*	Rt 1 Box 315 A Brinley	49715	1			CC	PBL			24	10	3	0	
007	Charles Stewart Mott Comm College Ms Patricia Markowicz, Assoc Dean *Chair's #: (810) 232-3271*	1401 E Court St Flint	48503	7			CC	PBL			Data reported w/AD Prog			
012	Delta College Mrs Louise Brentin. Chair *Chair's #: (517) 686-9500 Ext 9274*	University Center	48710	7			CC	PBL			Data reported w/AD prog			

School Code	Name of School, Director of Program, and Phone Number	Street Address / City or Town and Zip Code		Footnotes	Type of Program	NLNAC Accreditation as of January 31, 1999	Administrative Control	Financial Support (principal source)	Number of Months in Program	Educational Requirements for Entering Adult Program	Enrollments as of October 15, 1998	Admissions Aug. 1, 1997 - July 31, 1998	Graduations Aug. 1, 1997 - July 31, 1998	Fall Admissions Aug. 1, 1998 - Dec. 31, 1998
	MICHIGAN													
	- Continued													
036	Glen Oaks Comm College-Div Nsg Ed / Mrs Gail Brown, Dir / *Chair's #: (616) 467-9945 Ext 247*	62249 Shimmel Rd / Centreville	49032				CC	PBL			Publication withheld			
041	Gogebic Comm College / Ms Kathryn Encalada, Director / *Chair's #: (906) 932-4231 Ext 342*	E 4946 Jackson Rd / Ironwood	49938				CC	PBL	11	12	12	17	15	13
008	Grand Rapids Comm College / Mrs Marilyn Smidt, Dir / *Chair's #: (616) 234-4231*	143 Bostwick, NE / Grand Rapids	49502			A	CC	PBL	10	12	136	109	28	32
016	Grand Rapids Educ Center / Ms Margaret Palermo, Coord / *Chair's #: (616) 364-8464 Ext 46*	1750 Woolworth / Grand Rapids	49505	1			TCH	PBL			Publication withheld			
005	Great Lakes College / Mrs Barbara Carter, Dir / *Chair's #: (517) 835-4501 Ext 29*	3555 East Patrick Rd / Midland	48642				CC	PVT			Data reported w/AD prog			
018	Jackson Comm College / Ms Kathy Walsh, Chair / *Chair's #: (517) 787-0800 Ext 8515*	2111 Emmons Rd / Jackson	49201				CC	PBL			Publication withheld			
023	JTPA Sch of Practical Nursing / Ms Lula Johnson, Acting Dir / *Chair's #: (313) 596-7608*	735 Griswold / Detroit	48226			A	SEC	PBL	12	12	92	110	76	57
044	Kalamazoo Valley Comm College / Mrs Carol Roe, Director / *Chair's #: (616) 327-5365*	6767 West O Ave / Kalamazoo	49009	7			CC	PBL			Data reported w/AD prog			
006	Kellogg Comm College / Mrs Cynthia Sublett, Dir / *Chair's #: (616) 965-3931 Ext 2309*	450 North Ave / Battle Creek	49016				CC	PBL	9	12	14	27	20	15
043	Kirtland Comm College / Ms Karen Brown, Dir / *Chair's #: (517) 275-5121 Ext 298*	10775 N St Helen Rd / Roscommon	48653	7			CC	PBL			Publication withheld			
020	Lake Michigan College / Mrs Alice Rasmussen, Coord / *Chair's #: (616) 927-8100 Ext 5092*	2755 E Napier Ave / Benton Harbor	49022	7			CC	PBL			Data reported w/AD Prog			
004	Lansing Comm College / Dorothy Martin, Acting Dir / *Chair's #: (517) 483-1410*	419 N Capitol Ave / Lansing	48914	7			CC	PBL			Data reported w/AD Prog			
037	Mid-Michigan Comm College / Mrs Beth Sendre, Director / *Chair's #: (517) 386-6645*	1375 S Clare Ave / Harrison	48625	7			CC	PBL			Data reported w/AD Prog			

Explanation of footnotes on page x

School Code	Name of School, Director of Program, and Phone Number	Street Address / City or Town and Zip Code		Footnotes	Type of Program	NLNAC Accreditation as of January 31, 1999	Administrative Control	Financial Support (principal source)	Number of Months in Program	Educational Requirements for Entering Adult Program	Enrollments as of October 15, 1998	Admissions Aug. 1, 1997 - July 31, 1998	Graduations Aug. 1, 1997 - July 31, 1998	Fall Admissions Aug. 1, 1998 - Dec. 31, 1998
	MICHIGAN													
	- Continued													
035	Montcalm Comm College Ms Susan Wambach, Assoc Dean *Chair's #: (517) 328-1240*	Sidney	48885				CC	PBL			49	50	49	30
021	Muskegon County Comm College Mrs Darlene Collet, Director *Chair's #: (616) 777-0332*	221 S Quarterline Rd Muskegon	49443	7			CC	PBL			Data Reported w/AD Prog			
009	Northern Michigan Univ-PN Dept Ms Cheryl Karvonen, Dept Dir *Chair's #: (906) 227-2640*	College Of Nursing Marquette	49855				COL	PBL	12	12	40	40	35	40
010	NW Michigan College-PN Ctr Mrs Laura Schmidt, Coord *Chair's #: (616) 922-1245*	1701 E Front St Traverse City	49686				CC	PBL	12	12	31	17	15	21
025	Oakland Comm College Ms Louise Jasinski, Interim Dean *Chair's #: (248) 360-3107*	7350 Cooley Lake Rd Waterford	48327				CC	PBL	12	12	20	18	34	18
027	Schoolcraft College Mrs Midge Carleton, Asst Dean *Chair's #: (734) 462-4400 Ext 5226*	18600 Haggerty Rd Livonia	48151				CC	PBL			Publication withheld			
034	Southwestern Michigan Coll Miss Marilouise Hagenberg, Dean *Chair's #: (616) 782-1237*	58900 Cherry Grove Rd Dowagiac	49047	7			CC	PBL			Data reported w/AD prog			
015	St Clair Co Comm College Mrs Susan J Meeker, Dir *Chair's #: (810) 989-5680*	323 Erie St PO Box 5015 Port Huron	48061				CC	PBL	12	12	97	80	73	81
038	West Shore Comm College Mrs Patricia Collins, Dir *Chair's #: (616) 845-6211 Ext 3518*	PO Box 277 Scottville	49454				CC	PBL			28	30	24	30
	MINNESOTA													
	26 Programs in 26 Schools													
024	Alexandria Tech College Mrs Jola Amundsen, Director *Chair's #: (320) 762-4447*	1601 Jefferson St Alexandria	56308				TCH	PBL			62	64	57	32
032	Anoka-Hennepin Tech College Ms Glenda Jensen, Dir *Chair's #: (612) 576-4959*	1355 W Hwy 10 Anoka	55303			A	TCH	PBL			Publication withheld			
018	Central Lake College Mrs Lois Fieldings, Dir *Chair's #: (218) 828-2525*	501 W College Dr Brainerd	56401				COL	PBL	10	12	58	60	58	58

Explanation of footnotes on page x

MINNESOTA

- Continued

School Code	Name of School, Director of Program, and Phone Number	Street Address / City or Town and Zip Code	Footnotes	Type of Program	NLNAC Accreditation as of January 31, 1999	Administrative Control	Financial Support (principal source)	Number of Months in Program	Educational Requirements for Entering Adult Program	Enrollments as of October 15, 1998	Admissions Aug. 1, 1997 - July 31, 1998	Graduations Aug. 1, 1997 - July 31, 1998	Fall Admissions Aug. 1, 1998 - Dec. 31, 1998
040	Dakota County Tech College-PN Prog Ms Meri Beth Kennedy, Dir *Chair's #: (651) 423-8311*	1300 145th St East Rosemount 55068			A	TCH	PBL	18	12	144	145	57	36
027	Fergus Falls Comm College Mrs Donna Quam, Coord *Chair's #: (218) 739-7500 Ext 7546*	1414 College Way Fergus Falls 56537				CC	PBL	9	12	48	30	23	48
039	Hennepin Tech College Ms Anne Cassens, Dir *Chair's #: (612) 550-3166*	9200 Flying Cloud Dr Eden Prairie 55347	HSE			TCH TCH	PBL PBL			Publication withheld			
026	Itasca Comm College Ms Charlene Sawyer, Director *Chair's #: (218) 327-4469*	1851 Hwy 169 E Grand Rapids 55744				CC	PBL	15	12	23	31	31	26
002	Lake Superior Coll Ms Carleen Ronchetti, Dir *Chair's #: (218) 733-7635*	2101 Trinity Rd Duluth 55811				CC	PBL	13	12	267	41	58	42
035	Mesabi Range Comm and Tech Colleg Mrs Josephine Eluff, Dir *Chair's #: (218) 744-7457*	1100 Industrial Pk Dr Eveleth 55734				TCH	PBL	18	12	34	50	19	0
006	Minneapolis Comm Tech Coll Ms Jane Foote, Dir *Chair's #: (612) 341-7063*	1501 Hennepin Ave So Minneapolis 55403			A	CC	PBL	15	12	143	110	66	30
044	Minnesota West Comm And Tech Coll Mrs Jacqueline Otkin, Director *Chair's #: (507) 825-4054 Ext 237*	Box 250 Pipestone 56164				TCH	PBL			Publication withheld			
037	Minnesota West Comm and Tech Coll Ms Kathi Haberman, Dir *Chair's #: (507) 372-3443*	1450 Collegeway Worthington 56187				CC	PBL	13	12	26	28	24	24
013	Northland Comm And Tech Coll Ms Debra Filer, Dean *Chair's #: (218) 681-0841*	1101 Hwy One E Thief River Falls 56701	HS HSE			CC CC CC	PBL PBL PBL	12 12 12	12 12 12	108 2	95 6	62 0	64 4
031	Northwest Tech Coll Ms LeVon Strong, Director *Chair's #: (218) 847-1341 Ext 316*	900 Highway 34 E Detroit Lakes 56501				TCH	PBL			Publication withheld			
029	Northwest Tech Coll Mrs Karen Sollom, Director *Chair's #: (218) 755-4270*	905 Grant Ave SE Bemidji 56601				TCH	PBL			Publication withheld			
038	Northwest Tech College Ms Mary Wiersma, Dir *Chair's #: (218) 773-4556*	2022 Central Ave NE East Grand Forks 56721				TCH	PBL			Publication withheld			

Explanation of footnotes on page x

School Code	Name of School, Director of Program, and Phone Number	Street Address City or Town and Zip Code		Footnotes	Type of Program	NLNAC Accreditation as of January 31, 1999	Administrative Control	Financial Support (principal source)	Number of Months in Program	Educational Requirements for Entering Adult Program	Enrollments as of October 15, 1998	Admissions Aug. 1, 1997 - July 31, 1998	Graduations Aug. 1, 1997 - July 31, 1998	Fall Admissions Aug. 1, 1998 - Dec. 31, 1998
	MINNESOTA													
	- Continued													
042	Rainy River Comm Coll-PN Prog Mrs Judy Junker, Director *Chair's #: (218) 285-7722*	1501 Highway 71 Internatl Falls	56649				CC	PBL			Publication withheld			
014	Red Wing-Winona Tech Coll Ms Marsha Edblom Zich, Dir *Chair's #: (651) 385-6300 Ext 6371*	308 Pioneer Rd Red Wing	55066				CC	PBL			74	109	28	31
012	Red Wing-Winona Tech Coll Ms Laurie Becker, Director *Chair's #: (507) 453-2635*	110 Galewski Dr Winona	55987		HSE		TCH TCH	PBL PBL			Publication withheld			
011	Ridgewater College Ms Lynn Johnson, Dir *Chair's #: (320) 231-6034*	2101 15th Ave NW Box 1097 Willmar	56201			A	TCH	PBL	12	12	113	128	60	92
004	Riverland Comm Coll Ms Patricia Parson, Dir *Chair's #: (507) 453-0826*	1900 Eighth Ave NW Austin	55912				CC	PBL			Publication withheld			
015	Rochester Comm And Tech Coll Ms Lorna Schmidt, Dir *Chair's #: (507) 280-3161*	851 30th Ave SE Rochester	55904			A	CC	PBL	18	12	40	38	28	58
034	South Central Tech Coll Mrs Phyllis Wegner, Dir *Chair's #: (507) 389-7368*	1920 Lee Blvd N Mankato	56002		HS		TCH TCH	PBL PBL			Publication withheld			
005	South Central Tech Coll Ms Phyllis Wegner, Dir *Chair's #: (507) 332-5801*	1225 Third St SW Faribault	55021		HS		TCH TCH	PBL PBL	12	12 12	54 0	62 0	25 0	0 30
030	St Cloud Tech College PN Prog Mrs Gayle Melberg, Dean *Chair's #: (320) 654-5010*	1540 Northway Dr St Cloud	56303			A	TCH	PBL	18	12	83	100	72	50
036	St Paul Tech College PN Prog Dr Marilyn Krasowski, Dir *Chair's #: (612) 221-1413*	235 Marshall Ave St Paul	55102			A	TCH	PBL	0	12	180	145	62	80
	MISSISSIPPI													
	29 Programs in 15 Schools													
900	Coahoma Comm Coll Mr Jerone Shaw, Coord *Chair's #: (601) 627-2571 Ext 291*	Rt 1 Box 616 Clarksdale	38614	6			CC	PBL			Publication withheld			
047	Copiah-Lincoln Comm College (2 Brchs) Mr Louis Dugas, Dean *Chair's #: (601) 643-8322*	Box 649 Wesson	39191				CC	PBL	12	12	48	57	30	54

Explanation of footnotes on page x

School Code	Name of School, Director of Program, and Phone Number	Street Address, City or Town and Zip Code		Footnotes	Type of Program	NLNAC Accreditation as of January 31, 1999	Administrative Control	Financial Support (principal source)	Number of Months in Program	Educational Requirements for Entering Adult Program	Enrollments as of October 15, 1998	Admissions Aug. 1, 1997 - July 31, 1998	Graduations Aug. 1, 1997 - July 31, 1998	Fall Admissions Aug. 1, 1998 - Dec. 31, 1998
	MISSISSIPPI – Continued													
081	East Central Comm College, Mr John Addock, Dir, Chair's #: (601) 635-3237 Ext 211	PO Box 129, Decatur	39327				CC	PBL			Publication withheld			
050	East MS Comm College (2 Branches), Mrs Denise Tennison, Chair, Chair's #: (601) 243-1900	-Box 100, Mayhew	39753				CC	PVT			Publication withheld			
012	Hinds Comm College (2 Branches), Ms Dolores Gadner, Chair, Chair's #: (601) 372-6507	1750 Chadwick Dr, Jackson	39204				TCH	PBL			118	194	99	120
046	Holmes Comm College (3 Branches), Mrs Gail Caraway, Director, Chair's #: (601) 472-9114	Box 369, Goodman	39079				CC	PBL			Publication withheld			
032	Itawamba Comm College, Ms Treny Guntharp, Dir, Chair's #: (601) 620-5000 Ext 451	2176 East Eason Blvd, Tupelo	38801				TCH	PBL			24	25	18	25
091	Jones County Junior College, Ms Sandra Waldrup, Dir, Chair's #: (601) 477-4100	900 E Court St, Ellisville	39437				CC	PBL	12	12	75	84	68	44
099	Meridian Comm College, Ms Rowena Saucier, Coord, Chair's #: (601) 484-8241	910 Hwy 19 N, Meridian	39302			A	CC	PBL	12	12	47	55	43	29
090	MS Delta Comm College (4 Branches), Dr Martha Heffner, Asst Dean, Chair's #: (601) 246-6322	Box 668, Moorhead	39761				CC	PBL			Publication withheld			
096	MS Gulf Coast Comm College (3 Brchs), Dr Judith Benvenutti, Coord, Chair's #: (601) 928-6335	609 Silverun Rd, Perkinston	39573	7		A	CC	PBL	12	12	72	94	51	96
044	NE Mississippi Comm College, Mr Kenneth Pounders, Div Head, Chair's #: (601) 728-7751	101 Cunningham Blvd, Booneville	38829				CC	PBL			Publication withheld			
089	NW Mississippi Comm Coll (4 Branche), Mr Joe Broadway, Director, Chair's #: (601) 562-3200	51 N Box 7045, Senatobia	38668				CC	PBL			Publication withheld			
045	Pearl River Comm College (2 Brchs), Ms Edith Royse, Chair, Chair's #: (601) 795-6801	101 Hwy 11 North, Poplarville	39470				CC	PBL			Publication withheld			
021	SW Mississippi Comm Coll, Mrs Frances Morris, Coord, Chair's #: (601) 276-2000 Ext 3851	College Dr, Summit	39666				TCH	PBL	12	12	37	38	31	38

MISSOURI

42 Programs in 42 Schools

School Code	Name of School, Director of Program, and Phone Number	Street Address City or Town and Zip Code	Footnotes	Type of Program	NLNAC Accreditation as of January 31, 1999	Administrative Control	Financial Support (principal source)	Number of Months in Program	Educational Requirements for Entering Adult Program	Enrollments as of October 15, 1998	Admissions Aug. 1, 1997 - July 31, 1998	Graduations Aug. 1, 1997 - July 31, 1998	Fall Admissions Aug. 1, 1998 - Dec. 31, 1998
016	Applied Technology Services/W County Mrs Maudie Streetman, Coord *Chair's #: (314) 579-4805*	13480 South Outer 40 Hwy Chesterfield 63017				TCH	PBL	12	12	29	34	28	19
044	Boonslick Area Voc-Tech School Mrs Janie Higgins, Coord *Chair's #: (660) 882-5306*	1694 Ashley Rd Boonville 65233				TCH	PVT	12	12	21	27	24	21
043	Cape Girardeau Area Voc-Tech Sch Mrs C Eaker-Kranawetter, Coord *Chair's #: (573) 334-0826 Ext 26*	301 N Clark Cape Girardeau 63701				TCH	PBL	12	12	24	25	18	25
037	Cass Career Center Mrs Elaine Boyd, Coord *Chair's #: (816) 380-3253*	1600 East Elm Harrisonville 64701	1			TCH	PBL	11	12	18	0	0	21
011	Columbia Public Schs-PN Program Mrs Sharon Taylor, Asst Dir *Chair's #: (573) 886-2276*	500 Strawn Rd Columbia 65203			A	TCH	PBL			60	62	45	32
046	Gibson AVTS Mrs Joann Chalfant, Coord *Chair's #: (417) 272-3459*	PO Box 169 Reeds Spring 65737				TCH	PBL	12	12	28	32	27	34
017	Hannibal Public Sch of PN Mrs Gwenda Pollard, Coord *Chair's #: (573) 221-4430 Ext 182*	4550 McMasters Ave Hannibal 63401				TCH	PBL	12	12	24	24	15	25
036	Jefferson College Ms Michele Soest, Director *Chair's #: (314) 789-3000 Ext 409*	1000 Viking Dr Hillsboro 63050			 HS	CC CC	PBL PBL	10	12 12	41 0	52 0	45 0	41 0
041	Kennett AVTS Mrs Brigitte Thiele, Coord *Chair's #: (573) 717-1123*	1400 W Washington Kennett 63857				TCH	PBL	12	12	17	21	17	20
024	Kirksville ATC Mrs Sherry Willis, Coord *Chair's #: (660) 626-1470*	1103 S Cottage Grove Kirksville 63501				TCH	PBL	12	12	24	24	22	25
032	Lex La-Ray Technical Center Ms Bernice Wagner, Coord *Chair's #: (660) 259-2264*	2323 High School Dr Lexington 64067				TCH	PBL			27	28	20	27
018	Mineral Area College, The Prog in PN Mrs Lana Harris, Coord *Chair's #: (573) 431-4593 Ext 276*	PO Box 1000 Park Hills 63601				CC	PBL			24	24	16	25
035	Moberly Area Comm Coll Ms Ruth Jones, Dir *Chair's #: (573) 581-1925*	1320 Paris Rd Mexico 65265				CC	PBL			Publication withheld			

School Code	Name of School, Director of Program, and Phone Number	Street Address City or Town and Zip Code		Footnotes	Type of Program	NLNAC Accreditation as of January 31, 1999	Administrative Control	Financial Support (principal source)	Number of Months in Program	Educational Requirements for Entering Adult Program	Enrollments as of October 15, 1998	Admissions Aug. 1, 1997 - July 31, 1998	Graduations Aug. 1, 1997 - July 31, 1998	Fall Admissions Aug. 1, 1998 - Dec. 31, 1998
	MISSOURI													
	- Continued													
027	Moberly Area Comm College Ms Terry Bichsel, Coord *Chair's #: (660) 263-4110 Ext 251*	101 College Ave Moberly	65270	1			CC	PBL	12	12	18	21	19	0
021	N S Hillyard Tech Sch Ms Jane Manion, Coord *Chair's #: (816) 671-4170 Ext 26*	3434 Faraon St St Joseph	64506				TCH	PBL			23	25	24	24
023	Nevada Regional Tech Center Ms Rebecca Householder, Admin *Chair's #: (417) 448-2016*	2015 N West St Nevada	64772				SEC	PBL	12	12	25	30	25	29
015	Nichols Career Ctr Mrs Patricia Jentsch, Coord *Chair's #: (573) 659-3110*	609 Union St Jefferson City	65101	A			TCH	PBL	12	12	27	34	22	28
020	North Central MO College Ms Patricia Dixon, Assoc Dean *Chair's #: (800) 880-6180 Ext 0310*	1301 E Main St Trenton	64683				CC	PBL	12	12	41	64	41	45
049	Northland Career Ctr AVTS Mrs Betty Boles, Coord *Chair's #: (816) 858-5505 Ext 21*	1801 Branch PO Box 1700 Platte City	64079				TCH	PBL			29	29	24	29
031	Northwest Technical Sch Ms Trudith S Dorrel, Coord *Chair's #: (660) 562-4139*	1515 South Munn Maryville	64468				TCH	PBL	11	12	21	25	20	25
012	Ozarks Tech Comm Coll Mrs Sandra Richardson, Dean *Chair's #: (417) 895-7149*	PO Box 5958 Springfield	65801				CC	PBL	12	12	39	35	44	27
003	Penn Valley Comm College Ms Mattie Eley, Interim Coord *Chair's #: (816) 482-5070*	2700 E 18th St Kansas City	64127	A			CC	PBL			65	49	32	50
042	Pike/Lincoln Tech Center Mrs Gail Branstetter, Coord *Chair's #: (573) 485-2900 Ext 0011*	430 VoTech Rd P.O.Box 38 Eolia	63344				TCH	PBL	12	12	23	11	8	24
007	Poplar Bluff Sch Dist, PN Prog Ms Patricia Markowic, Assoc Dean *Chair's #: (810) 785-6867*	3203 Oak Grove Rd Poplar Bluff	63901	7			TCH	PBL			Data Reported w/Adprog			
026	Rolla Tech Inst Mrs Pati Cox, Coord *Chair's #: (573) 364-3726 Ext 130*	1304 E 10th St Rolla	65401				TCH	PBL			Publication withheld			
030	Saline Co Career Center Mrs Stefanie Sauble, Admin *Chair's #: (660) 886-6958*	900 W Vest Marshall	65340				TCH	PBL			Publication withheld			

Explanation of footnotes on page x

School Code	Name of School, Director of Program, and Phone Number	Street Address City or Town and Zip Code		Footnotes	Type of Program	NLNAC Accreditation as of January 31, 1999	Administrative Control	Financial Support (principal source)	Number of Months in Program	Educational Requirements for Entering Adult Program	Enrollments as of October 15, 1998	Admissions Aug. 1, 1997 - July 31, 1998	Graduations Aug. 1, 1997 - July 31, 1998	Fall Admissions Aug. 1, 1998 - Dec. 31, 1998
	MISSOURI													
	- Continued													
901	Sanford Brown Coll Ms Vickie Baker-Janis, Dir *Chair's #: (314) 949-2620*	3555 Franks Dr St Charles	63301				TCH	PVT			Publication withheld			
900	Sanford Brown Coll Ms Kathy Sanquinet, Coord *Chair's #: (314) 822-8252*	12006 Manchester Rd St Louis	63131				TCH	PVT			Publication withheld			
008	Sanford Brown Coll Ms Cheryl Hendricks Scott, Dir *Chair's #: (816) 472-7400*	520 E 19th Ave N Kansas City	64116				TCH	PVT			Publication withheld			
010	School Dist of Joplin R-VIII Ms Joyce O'Malley, Coord *Chair's #: (417) 659-4403*	3950 East Newman Joplin	64804				TCH	PBL	12	12	49	54	39	26
022	Sikeston Public Schs (2 Branches) Mrs Pat Elledge, Coord *Chair's #: (573) 472-8887*	1002 Virginia Sikeston	63801		A		TCH	PBL	11	12	54	50	37	0
033	South Central AVTS Ms Marlene Martensen, Admin *Chair's #: (417) 256-6150 Ext 211*	613 W First St West Plains	65775				TCH	PBL	12	12	36	30	26	10
048	St Charles Co Comm College Ms Russlyn St John, Coord *Chair's #: (314) 922-8280*	4601 Mid River Mall Dr St Peters	63376				CC	PBL	14	12	12	14	14	0
002	St Louis Bd of Education PN Ms Mitzi Bryant, Coord *Chair's #: (314) 781-1322 Ext 250*	3815 McCausland Ave St Louis	63109				TCH	PBL			Publication withheld			
050	St Louis Coll of Hlth Career Mrs Deborah Goldseder, Dir *Chair's #: (314) 652-0300*	4484 West Pine Blvd St Louis	63108				TCH	PVT			Publication withheld			
006	St Louis Coll of Hlth Career Mrs Deborah Goldseder, Dir *Chair's #: (314) 845-6100*	4044 Butler Hill Rd St Louis	63129	1			TCH	PVT			Publication withheld			
028	State Fair Comm College Ms Leora Bremer, Coord *Chair's #: (660) 530-5815 Ext 228*	3201 W 16th St Sedalia	65301	1			CC	PBL			30	34	34	30
004	Tri County Tech Sch Mrs Susan Green, Coord *Chair's #: (573) 392-8066*	2nd & Pine St Eldon	65026				TCH	PBL	12	12	19	25	21	0
038	Warrensburg AVTS Mrs Marcile R Lewis, Coord *Chair's #: (660) 747-2283*	205 S Ridgeview Dr Warrensburg	64093				TCH	PBL	12	12	29	30	23	30

Explanation of footnotes on page x

School Code	Name of School, Director of Program, and Phone Number	Street Address, City or Town and Zip Code	Footnotes	Type of Program	NLNAC Accreditation as of January 31, 1999	Administrative Control	Financial Support (principal source)	Number of Months in Program	Educational Requirements for Entering Adult Program	Enrollments as of October 15, 1998	Admissions Aug. 1, 1997 - July 31, 1998	Graduations Aug. 1, 1997 - July 31, 1998	Fall Admissions Aug. 1, 1998 - Dec. 31, 1998
	MISSOURI **- Continued**												
034	Washington School of PN Mrs Christie Gildehaus, Coord *Chair's #: (314) 239-7777*	550 East Eleventh St Washington 63090				TCH	PVT	11	12	27	22	24	29
040	Waynesville Tech Academy Mrs Glenda Cole, Coord *Chair's #: (573) 774-6584*	810 Roosevelt St Waynesville 65583				TCH	PBL	12	12	29	30	25	31
	MONTANA **5 Programs in 5 Schools**												
010	Helena College of Technology Ms Linda McDonlad, Dir *Chair's #: (406) 444-1223*	2300 Poplar St Helena 59601				TCH	PBL			Publication withheld			
011	Montana State Univ-Billings Coll of Tec Dr Audrey Conner Rosberg, Dir *Chair's #: (406) 656-4445 Ext 150*	3803 Central Ave Billings 59102				CC	PBL	24	12	64	84	41	42
012	Montana Tech/Coll of Technology Mrs Karen Vandaveer, Director *Chair's #: (406) 496-3722*	Basin Creek Rd Butte 59701				TCH	PBL	18	12	60	24	20	14
004	MSU College of Technology Ms Connie MacKay, Dir *Chair's #: (406) 771-4352*	2100 16th Ave South Great Falls 59405				TCH	PBL	18	12	30	28	19	15
003	Univ of Montana Coll of Tech Ms Margaret A Wafstet, Dir *Chair's #: (406) 243-7864*	909 South Ave, W Missoula 59801				CC	PBL	16	12	55	76	40	36
	NEBRASKA **8 Programs in 7 Schools**												
006	Central Comm College (3 Branches) Mrs Linda Walline, Assoc Dean *Chair's #: (308) 389-6456*	PO Box 4903 3134 W Hwy 34 Grand Island 68502				TCH	PBL			82	99	65	63
001	Metropolitan Comm College Dr Janice T Adkins, Chair *Chair's #: (402) 457-2367*	PO Box 3777 Omaha 68103				CC	PBL	15	12	26	30	18	30
008	Mid-Plains Comm College Mrs Pauline Shahan, Dept Head *Chair's #: (308) 532-8740 Ext 322*	1101 Hallgan Dr North Platte 69101	A			CC	PBL	12	12	34	44	36	27
005	Northeast Comm College Mrs Anita Brenneman, Chair *Chair's #: (402) 644-0444 Ext 4444*	801 E Benjamin Ave Box 469 Norfolk 68702				CC	PBL	12	12	37	51	28	19
004	SE Nebraska Comm College-Lincoln Ms Iris Winkelhake, Chair *Chair's #: (402) 437-2765*	8800 0 St Lincoln 68520	A			CC	PBL	0	12	49	62	47	30

Explanation of footnotes on page x

School Code	Name of School, Director of Program, and Phone Number	Street Address / City or Town and Zip Code	Footnotes	Type of Program	NLNAC Accreditation as of January 31, 1999	Administrative Control	Financial Support (principal source)	Number of Months in Program	Educational Requirements for Entering Adult Program	Enrollments as of October 15, 1998	Admissions Aug. 1, 1997 - July 31, 1998	Graduations Aug. 1, 1997 - July 31, 1998	Fall Admissions Aug. 1, 1998 - Dec. 31, 1998
	NEBRASKA												
	- Continued												
009	Southeast Comm College-Beatrice Cam Mrs Crystal Higgins, Chair *Chair's #: (402) 228-3468 Ext 264*	Box 35A Route 2 Beatrice 68310			A	CC	PBL	12	12	37	53	35	9
003	Western Nebraska Comm College (2 Brc Ms Anne Hippe, Chair *Chair's #: (308) 635-6060 Ext 6181*	1601 East 27th ST Scottsbluff 69361			A	CC	PBL	0	12	29	33	24	37
	NEVADA												
	1 Program in 1 School												
010	W Nevada Comm College-Carson City Ms Mildred Wade, Dir *Chair's #: (775) 887-3176*	2201 W College Parkway Carson City 89701	7			CC	PBL			Data reported w/AD Prog			
	NEW HAMPSHIRE												
	2 Programs in 2 Schools												
006	New Hampshire Comm Tech Dr Susan Henderson, Chair *Chair's #: (603) 542-7744 Ext 2739*	One College Dr RR#3 Box 550 Claremont 03743				CC	PBL	14	12	69	34	30	69
004	St Joseph Sch of Practical Nsg Ms Barbara Provencher, Dir *Chair's #: (603) 594-2566*	5 Woodward Ave Nashua 03060			A	HSP	PVT	17	12	101	75	52	51
	NEW JERSEY												
	22 Programs in 22 Schools												
029	Atlantic County Voc Sch Ms Rosalie G Mocco, Coord *Chair's #: (609) 625-2249 Ext 1315*	5080 Atlantic Ave Mays Landing 08330				TCH	PBL	11	12	26	33	26	28
022	Burlington Co Voc and Tech Schs Mrs Alice Sinclair, Supv *Chair's #: (609) 654-0200 Ext 426*	Medford Campus Hawkins Rd Medford 08055				TCH	PBL	11	12	20	0	12	20
027	Camden Bd of Education Ms Danna Beverly, Coord *Chair's #: (609) 966-2479*	1656 Kaighns Ave Camden 08103				SEC	PBL	18	12	48	24	18	30
004	Camden Co Voc Tech Sch Ms J Clark, Coord *Chair's #: (856) 767-7000 Ext 5540*	343 Berlin Cross Keys Rd Sicklerville 08081				TCH	PBL			Publication withheld			
021	Cape May County Tech Sch Mr Rusty Miller, Dir *Chair's #: (609) 465-2161 Ext 645*	188 Crest Haven Rd Cape May C H 08210				TCH	PBL	11	12	16	20	20	20
035	Cumberland County Tech Educ Center Mrs Priscilla Meyers, Coord *Chair's #: (609) 451-9000 Ext 245*	601 Bridgeton Ave Bridgeton 08302				TCH	PBL	12	12	20	22	20	24

Explanation of footnotes on page x

School Code	Name of School, Director of Program, and Phone Number	Street Address City or Town and Zip Code	Footnotes	Type of Program	NLNAC Accreditation as of January 31, 1999	Administrative Control	Financial Support (principal source)	Number of Months in Program	Educational Requirements for Entering Adult Program	Enrollments as of October 15, 1998	Admissions Aug. 1, 1997 - July 31, 1998	Graduations Aug. 1, 1997 - July 31, 1998	Fall Admissions Aug. 1, 1998 - Dec. 31, 1998
	NEW JERSEY												
	- Continued												
001	Essex Co Tech Careers Ctr Mrs Loraine San Roman, Coord *Chair's #: (973) 622-1100 Ext 349*	91 W Market St Newark 07103				TCH	PBL	12	12	27	31	23	28
044	Gloucester Co Voc School Ms Patricia A Mulutzie, Coord *Chair's #: (609) 468-1445 Ext 2330*	PO Box 800 Tanyard Rd Sewell 08080				TCH	PBL	12	12	16	20	22	18
038	Holy Name Hosp Sr Claire Tynan, Senior Vice Pres *Chair's #: (201) 833-3008*	690 Teaneck Rd Teaneck 07666				HSP	PVT	12	12	29	25	23	27
026	Hudson County Voc Sch Mrs Carol Cruden, Dir *Chair's #: (201) 413-5900*	W 30th St Bayonne 07002				TCH	PBL		Publication withheld				
034	Mercer County Technical School Mrs V Clevenger, Supv *Chair's #: (609) 587-7640*	1070 Klockner Rd Trenton 08619				TCH	PBL	12	12	58	44	28	58
039	Middlesex Co V-T Sch of PN (4 Brchs) Mrs Joan McNulty, Director *Chair's #: (732) 613-9201*	112 Rues Ln Box 1070 East Brunswick 08816				TCH	PBL	11	12	169	136	132	83
015	Monmouth County Voc Sch Dist Mrs Iris Arbeitman, Dir *Chair's #: (732) 922-9272*	185 State Route 36 West Long Branch 07764				TCH	PBL		Publication withheld				
037	Morris Co Voc Sch Mr Gene Polles, Director *Chair's #: (973) 627-4600 Ext 232*	400 E Main St Denville 07834				TCH	PBL	12	12	12	19	11	19
016	Ocean County Voc Tech Sch Mrs Barbara Haines, Vice Principal *Chair's #: (732) 473-3139*	1299 Old Freehold Rd Toms River 08753				TCH	PBL		Publication withheld				
007	Passaic Co Tech and Voc HS Ms Athena Fitzgerald, Coord *Chair's #: (973) 628-9208*	1006 Hamburg Turnpike Wayne 07470				TCH	PBL	11	12	19	25	19	22
013	Salem Comm College Mrs Alice Gloor, Dir *Chair's #: (609) 351-2648*	Carneys Point 08069				CC	PBL	12	12	12	15	8	12
018	Somerset Co Voc-Tech Sch Mrs Nanette Craig, Supv *Chair's #: (908) 526-8900 Ext 7235*	PO Box 6350 Bridgewater 08807				TCH	PBL		Publication withheld				
019	Sussex County Voc-Tech Schs Mrs Maureen S Howard, Dir *Chair's #: (973) 383-6700 Ext 222*	105 North Church Rd Sparta 07871				TCH	PBL	11	12	19	22	16	23

Explanation of footnotes on page x

School Code	Name of School, Director of Program, and Phone Number	Street Address / City or Town and Zip Code		Footnotes	Type of Program	NLNAC Accreditation as of January 31, 1999	Administrative Control	Financial Support (principal source)	Number of Months in Program	Educational Requirements for Entering Adult Program	Enrollments as of October 15, 1998	Admissions Aug. 1, 1997 - July 31, 1998	Graduations Aug. 1, 1997 - July 31, 1998	Fall Admissions Aug. 1, 1998 - Dec. 31, 1998
	NEW JERSEY													
	- Continued													
023	Union County College Miss Ellen Boddie, Dir *Chair's #: (908) 965-6088 Ext 6088*	12-24 W Jersey St Elizabeth	07202			A	CC	PBL			Publication withheld			
028	Vineland Adult Center Mrs Gloria Rochetti, Director *Chair's #: (609) 794-6943*	48 Landis Ave Vineland	08360				SEC	PBL			28	35	32	34
020	Warren Co Voc Sch and Tech Inst Mr Frank Mancuso, Dir *Chair's #: (908) 689-0122 Ext 14*	Rd 1, Box 168A Washington	07882				TCH	PBL			Publication withheld			
	NEW MEXICO													
	8 Programs in 8 Schools													
020	Albuquerque Public Schs of PN Mrs Nancy Hatfield, Dept Chair *Chair's #: (505) 247-3658 Ext 0038*	807 Mountain Rd NE Albuquerque	87102		HS	A A	SEC SEC	PBL PBL	20	10	0 64	0 75	0 25	0 70
004	Albuquerque TVI Mrs Patricia Stephens, Director *Chair's #: (505) 224-4141*	525 Buena Vista SE Albuquerque	87106			A	CC	PBL	12	12	18	22	23	0
017	Clovis Comm Coll Mrs Ione Wood, Director *Chair's #: (505) 769-4975*	417 Schepps Blvd Clovis	88101				CC	PBL	0	12	38	80	64	39
010	Eastern New Mexico Univ at Roswell Ms Tammy Bennett, Dir *Chair's #: (505) 624-7237*	PO Box 6000 Roswell	88201	7			CC	PBL			Data reported w/Ad prog			
014	Luna Voc Tech Inst Mrs Beatrice Hurtado, Interim Dir *Chair's #: (505) 454-2524*	PO Box 1510 Las Vegas	87701	7			CC	PBL	9	12	26	22	16	26
009	New Mexico Jr College Mr Steven M Davis, Director *Chair's #: (505) 392-5714*	5317 Lovington Highway Hobbs	88240	7			CC	PBL			Data reported w/AD prog			
018	New Mexico State Univ Ms Sharon Souter, Dir *Chair's #: (505) 234-9301*	1500 University Dr Carlsbad	88220	7			CC	PBL			Data reported w/AD prog			
002	Northern New Mexico Comm College Ms Ramona Gonzales, Dir *Chair's #: (505) 747-2209*	921 Paseo de Onate Espanola	87532	7			CC	PBL			Data reported w/AD Prog			
	NEW YORK													
	113 Programs in 52 Schools													
011	Albany-Schoharie-Schenectady BOCES Ms Joanne O'Brien, Coord *Chair's #: (518) 456-9202*	1015 Watervliet-Shaker Rd Albany	12205		HS		TCH TCH	PVT PVT			Publication withheld			

Explanation of footnotes on page x

NEW YORK

- Continued

School Code	Name of School, Director of Program, and Phone Number	Street Address / City or Town and Zip Code	Footnotes	Type of Program	NLNAC Accreditation as of January 31, 1999	Administrative Control	Financial Support (principal source)	Number of Months in Program	Educational Requirements for Entering Adult Program	Enrollments as of October 15, 1998	Admissions Aug. 1, 1997 - July 31, 1998	Graduations Aug. 1, 1997 - July 31, 1998	Fall Admissions Aug. 1, 1998 - Dec. 31, 1998
902	Bronx Comm College Mrs Ellen R Hoist, Director *Chair's #: (718) 289-5420*	181 St University Ave Rm 408 Bronx 10453				CC	PVT	18	12	56	33	0	23
764	Broome-Tioga BOCES Mrs Annette Gould, Coord *Chair's #: (607) 786-8504*	435 Glenwood Rd Binghamton 13905				SEC	PBL	20	12	35	21	15	20
016	Buffalo Voc-Tech Ctr Mrs Kathleen Sorrentino, Admin *Chair's #: (716) 897-8108*	820 Northampton St Buffalo 14211		HSE		TCH TCH	PBL PBL	12 25	12 12	42 7	46 8	46 6	24 8
762	Catragus-Allgny-Wyomg-Erie BOCES Mrs Judith Barillo, Specialist *Chair's #: (716) 372-8293 Ext 217*	Windfall Rd, Box 424B Olean 14760		HSE		TCH TCH	PBL PBL	12 21	12 12	72 10	53 17	32 4	58 3
714	Cayuga/Onondaga BOCES Miss Patricia Kenny, Coord *Chair's #: (315) 253-0361 Ext 153*	5980 S St Rd Auburn 13021		HSE		TCH TCH	PBL PBL	10 17	12 12	13 12	19 20	16 3	0 6
098	Champlain Valley Tech Educ Cereer Ce Mrs Joan Rice, Coord *Chair's #: (518) 561-0100 Ext 248*	PO Box 455 Plattsburgh 12901				TCH	PBL			96	38	23	38
064	Clara Barton HS for Hlth Profs Mrs Julia Blair, Dir *Chair's #: (718) 636-4900 Ext 263*	901 Classon Ave Brooklyn 11225		HS		SEC SEC	PBL PBL	22		0 47	0 29	0 24	0 29
711	Coopers Edu Center Mr Nile Heerman, Dir *Chair's #: (607) 962-3175 Ext 271*	One Vocational Dr. Painted Post 14870				TCH	PBL	10	12	45	41	29	55
091	Curtis HS-Secondary Prog Mrs Lynn Davis, Coord *Chair's #: (718) 273-7380 Ext 305*	105 Hamilton Ave Staten Island 10301		HS		SEC SEC	PBL PBL	22		0 39	0 32	0 11	0 18
027	Delaware Chen Mad BOCES Mrs Ann Marie Sullivan, Coord *Chair's #: (607) 335-1303 Ext 1303*	Rd # 3 PO Box 307 Norwich 13815				SEC	PBL			Publication withheld			
742	Delhi Coll of Tech Ms Mary J Giarrusso-Wilkin, Chair *Chair's #: (607) 746-4490*	Delhi 13753	7			CC	PBL			Data reported/AD prog			
715	Dutchess BOCES Mrs Margaret Muraca, Coord *Chair's #: (914) 486-8045*	Rd 1 Box 369A Salt Pt Turnpik Poughkeepsie 12601				TCH	PBL			Publication withheld			
093	Eastern Suffolk Sch for PN Mrs Carol Powell, Administrator *Chair's #: (516) 286-6591*	350 Martha Ave Bellport 11713		HSE	A A	TCH TCH	PVT PVT	18 18	12 12	220 70	120 60	164 0	110 70

School Code	Name of School, Director of Program, and Phone Number	Street Address / City or Town and Zip Code		Footnotes	Type of Program	NLNAC Accreditation as of January 31, 1999	Administrative Control	Financial Support (principal source)	Number of Months in Program	Educational Requirements for Entering Adult Program	Enrollments as of October 15, 1998	Admissions Aug. 1, 1997 - July 31, 1998	Graduations Aug. 1, 1997 - July 31, 1998	Fall Admissions Aug. 1, 1998 - Dec. 31, 1998
	NEW YORK - Continued													
744	Ed Opportunity Ctr, PN Prog / Mrs Margaret Walker, Admin / Chair's #: (716) 546-8660 Ext 234	305 Andrews St / Rochester	14604				CC	PBL	11	12	58	124	52	64
771	Erie 2 Cattaraugus, BOCES / Mrs Marie Beckstrom, Coord / Chair's #: (716) 366-3891	1020 Central Ave / Dunkirk	14048				TCH	PBL	10	12	66	64	49	66
044	Erie BOCES-First Supv Dist / Mrs Georgiann Dudek, Coord / Chair's #: (716) 821-7033	355 Harlem Rd / West Seneca	14224	HSE			TCH	PBL	0		99	98	87	62
							TCH	PBL			49	66	0	55
003	Genesse Livingston Steuben / Ms Carolyn Thomas, Coord / Chair's #: (716) 344-7793	8250 State Street Rd / Batavia	14020				TCH	PBL	10		20	27	24	24
710	Hamilton-Fulton Montgmry BOCES / Mrs Judith Gisondi, Coord / Chair's #: (518) 762-4633 Ext 124	212 Co Hwy 103 Box 665 / Johnstown	12095	HS			SEC	PBL	21	12	24	10	15	19
							SEC	PBL	21	12	5	8	0	1
705	Herkimer BOCES / Ms Karolyn Lado, Coord / Chair's #: (315) 867-2040	Gros Blvd / E Herkimer	13350				TCH	PBL	10	12	38	52	26	40
745	Hillcrest HS / Mrs L Dunworth, Asst Principal / Chair's #: (718) 658-5407 Ext 362	160-05 Highland Ave / Jamaica	11432	HS			SEC	PBL			0	0	0	0
							SEC	PBL	22		35	57	21	36
069	Isabella G Hart Sch-Rochester Gen Hosp / Mrs Nina Morris, Dir / Chair's #: (716) 922-1401	1425 Portland Ave / Rochester	14621			A	HSP	PVT	10	12	70	57	31	75
094	Jefferson-Lewis Co BOCES Prog / Mrs Diane Riddell, Coord / Chair's #: (315) 789-3410 Ext 308	Arsenal St, Rd 1 / Watertown	13601	HS			TCH	PBL	10	10	46	97	57	36
							TCH	PBL	22	10	68	120	25	44
718	Madison & Oneida BOCES PN Prog / Mrs Virginia Parrott, Coord / Chair's #: (315) 361-5800	Spring Rd / Verona	13478	HS			SEC	PBL	10		73	82	71	37
							SEC	PBL	22		10	7	16	10
017	Marion S Whelan Sch of Practical Nsg / Ms E Ann O'conner, Director / Chair's #: (315) 787-4003	196-198 North St / Geneva	14456			A	HSP	PVT	12	12	10	14	17	10
008	Medgar Evers Coll of CUNY / Ms Delores Casey, Coord / Chair's #: (212) 270-6442	1650 Bedford Ave / Brooklyn	11222				COL	PBL			Publication withheld			
738	Nassau BOCES / Mrs Eileen Brown, Coord / Chair's #: (516) 622-6901	1196 Prospect Ave / Westbury	11590			A	TCH	PBL	11	12	264	378	240	110
				HS		A	TCH	PBL	30	12	0	0	0	0
				HSE		A	TCH	PBL	16	12				

Explanation of footnotes on page x

School Code	Name of School, Director of Program, and Phone Number	Street Address City or Town and Zip Code	Footnotes	Type of Program	NLNAC Accreditation as of January 31, 1999	Administrative Control	Financial Support (principal source)	Number of Months in Program	Educational Requirements for Entering Adult Program	Enrollments as of October 15, 1998	Admissions Aug. 1, 1997 - July 31, 1998	Graduations Aug. 1, 1997 - July 31, 1998	Fall Admissions Aug. 1, 1998 - Dec. 31, 1998
	NEW YORK												
	- Continued												
900	Niagara Co Comm College-Nsg Educ Mrs Catherine Peuquet, Director Chair's #: (716) 731-3271 Ext 265	3111 Saunders Settlement Rd Sanborn 14132				CC	PBL	10	12	47	68	50	23
724	North Country Comm College Ms Penny Dieffenbach, Dir Chair's #: (518) 891-2915 Ext 302	20 Winona Ave Box 89 Saranac Lake 12983				CC	PBL	9	12	33	33	24	4
716	Oneida BOCES PN Prog Ms Mary Beth Piejko, Coord Chair's #: (315) 793-8642	Mid Settlement Rd-Box 70 New Hartford 13413	HS			SEC SEC	PBL PBL	22	10	0 12	0 14	0 14	0 13
765	Onondaga & Madison BOCES Mrs Allene Rossler, Coord Chair's #: (315) 453-4405	4500 Crown Rd Liverpool 13090				TCH	PBL			Publication withheld			
727	Orange Ulster BOCES Mr David Barker, Supv Chair's #: (914) 294-5431 Ext 231	Gibson Rd Goshen 10924				TCH	PBL			Publication withheld			
722	Orleans & Niagara BOCES Mrs Janet Taylor Cook, Dept Head Chair's #: (800) 836-7510 Ext 446	3181 Saunders Settlement Sanborn 14132	HS			SEC SEC	PBL PBL	22	12	8 19	5 21	5 18	10 19
046	Oswego BOCES Sch of PN HOC Mrs Elyse Skiles, Interim Supv Chair's #: (315) 963-4231	County Rt 64 Mexico 13114				SEC	PBL	10	12	19	48	45	20
725	Otsego Area Sch-Adult Mrs Sharyn Gibbons, Head Instructor Chair's #: (607) 286-7715	PO Box 57 Milford 13807				TCH	PBL	10	12	27	28	21	28
739	Putnam-Westchester BOCES Mr Kevin Hart, Director Chair's #: (914) 248-2450	200 Boces Dr Yorktown Hts 10598	HS			TCH TCH	PBL PBL	10 21	12 12	62 18	48 7	47 15	38 11
717	Rennselaer-Columbia BOCES Dr Frances Gaskin, Admin Chair's #: (518) 273-2264	97 Industrial Pk Rd Troy 12180	HS			TCH TCH	PBL PBL			Publication withheld			
059	Rockland BOCES Mr William Renella, Dir Chair's #: (914) 627-4700 Ext 4770	65 Parrot Rd West Nyack 10994	HS			TCH TCH	PBL PBL	19 19	12 12	48 4	56 7	33 3	45 4
001	Samaritan Hosp Sch of Nursing Ms Mary Harknett-Martin, Manager Chair's #: (518) 271-3285	Burdett Ave Troy 12180				HSP	PVT			Publication withheld			
747	Schuyler-Chemung Tioga BOCES Prog Mr Stan Swider, Supv Chair's #: (607) 739-3581 Ext 2398	459 Philo Rd Elmira 14903				TCH	PBL			60	60	50	0

Explanation of footnotes on page x

School Code	Name of School, Director of Program, and Phone Number	Street Address City or Town and Zip Code		Footnotes	Type of Program	NLNAC Accreditation as of January 31, 1999	Administrative Control	Financial Support (principal source)	Number of Months in Program	Educational Requirements for Entering Adult Program	Enrollments as of October 15, 1998	Admissions Aug. 1, 1997 - July 31, 1998	Graduations Aug. 1, 1997 - July 31, 1998	Fall Admissions Aug. 1, 1998 - Dec. 31, 1998
	NEW YORK													
	- Continued													
726	Southern-Westchester Prog of PN Mrs Barbara Biles, Coord *Chair's #: (914) 381-0853*	310 E Boston Post Rd Mamaroneck	10543				TCH	PBL			103	103	95	104
024	St Francis PN Program Mrs Faye Weir, Dir *Chair's #: (716) 375-7315*	2221 W State St Olean	14760			A	HSP	PVT	10	12	22	9	3	0
760	St Lawrence-Lewis BOCES Mrs Betty MacDonald, Coord *Chair's #: (315) 353-2194 Ext 301*	7231 State RTE 56 Norwood	13668	HS			TCH TCH	PBL PBL		12	58 30	38 23	36 41	36 30
013	Sullivan Co BOCES Mrs Kathleen Moran, Coord *Chair's #: (914) 292-7900 Ext 134*	85 Ferndale Looms Rd Liberty	12754	HSE			SEC SEC	PBL PBL			Publication withheld			
010	Syracuse Central Tech Voc Center Mrs Margaret O'Connor, Coord *Chair's #: (315) 435-4150*	258 E Adams St Syracuse	13202	HSE			TCH TCH	PBL PBL	10 10	12 12	51 26	0 18	41 1	28 14
081	Ulster BOCES Sch of PN Mrs Diane Davies, Admin *Chair's #: (914) 331-6680 Ext 232*	PO Box 601 Port Ewen	12466	HS			TCH TCH	PBL PBL	12 24	12 12	85 38	101 24	70 4	58 25
070	Voc Ed & Extn Bd-Nassau Co Sch Mrs Mary F Watson, Supervisor *Chair's #: (516) 572-1704*	899-A Jerusalem Ave Uniondale	11553			A	TCH	PVT	11	12	192	200	155	203
769	Wa-War'N-Hmltn Essex BOCES Mrs Sharon M Erbe, Coord *Chair's #: (518) 746-3428*	Dix Ave Hudson Falls	12839	HSE			TCH TCH	PBL PBL	11 17	12 12	31 56	22 44	14 26	32 36
023	Wayne-Finger Lakes BOCES (2 Branch Ms Beverlyann Zier, Admin *Chair's #: (315) 331-2346*	4440 E Ridge Rd Williamson	14589				TCH	PBL			42	81	55	60
766	Westchester Comm College Mrs Marie Cahill, Chair *Chair's #: (914) 785-6884*	75 Grasslands Rd Valhalla	10595				CC	PBL	11	12	37	54	32	0
055	Western Suffolk BOCES Mrs Kathleen Baker, Chairperson *Chair's #: (516) 261-3727 Ext 247*	Laurel Hill Rd Northport	11768	HSE		A A	TCH TCH	PBL PBL	10 20	12 12	112 20	106 20	82 2	63 22
	NORTH CAROLINA													
	28 Programs in 28 Schools													
047	Anson Comm College Mrs Sarah U Lee, Chair *Chair's #: (704) 272-7635 Ext 282*	PO Box 126 Polkton	28135				TCH	PBL	12	12	15	20	11	0

Explanation of footnotes on page x

School Code	Name of School, Director of Program, and Phone Number	Street Address / City or Town and Zip Code		Footnotes	Type of Program	NLNAC Accreditation as of January 31, 1999	Administrative Control	Financial Support (principal source)	Number of Months in Program	Educational Requirements for Entering Adult Program	Enrollments as of October 15, 1998	Admissions Aug. 1, 1997 - July 31, 1998	Graduations Aug. 1, 1997 - July 31, 1998	Fall Admissions Aug. 1, 1998 - Dec. 31, 1998
	NORTH CAROLINA													
	- Continued													
011	Asheville-Buncombe Tech Comm Colle Mrs Brenda Causey, Chair *Chair's #: (828) 254-1921 Ext 262*	340 Victoria Rd Asheville	28801				TCH	PBL	12	12	43	45	38	45
014	Beaufort Co Comm College Ms Carolyn Lee, Lead Instructor *Chair's #: (252) 946-6194 Ext 318*	PO Box 1069 Washington	27889				CC	PBL	12	12	18	20	15	20
901	Bladen Comm College Mrs Saundra Meares, Chair *Chair's #: (910) 862-2164 Ext 316*	PO Box 266 Dublin	28332				TCH	PBL	12	12	20	20	17	20
067	Brunswick Comm College Ms Connie Milliken, Director *Chair's #: (910) 755-7350*	PO Box 30 Supply	28462				CC	PBL	12	12	17	23	19	19
032	Cape Fear Comm College Ms Vinson Greene, Director *Chair's #: (910) 251-5190 Ext 8482*	411 N Front St Wilmington	28401				CC	PBL			Publication withheld			
035	Carteret Comm College Mrs Nancy McBride, Coord *Chair's #: (252) 247-6000 Ext 170*	3505 Arendell St Morehead City	28557				CC	PBL	12	12	19	23	19	19
069	Central Carolina Comm College Mrs Rhonda Evans, Chair *Chair's #: (919) 775-5401 Ext 281*	Route 1 Box 447-C Lillington	27546				CC	PBL			Publication withheld			
015	Cleveland Comm College Ms Katherine Jones, Dept Head *Chair's #: (704) 484-4001*	137 S Post Rd Shelby	28150				CC	PBL			Publication withheld			
036	Coastal Carolina Comm College Mrs Paula V Gribble, Chair *Chair's #: (910) 938-6269*	444 Western Blvd Jacksonville	28546				CC	PBL	12		11	18	17	0
013	Coll of the Albemarle Mrs Elizabeth Jones, Coord *Chair's #: (252) 335-0821 Ext 2289*	PO Box 2327 Elizabeth City	27906				CC	PBL	12	12	16	21	17	17
033	Craven Comm College Mrs Carolyn Jones, Director *Chair's #: (252) 638-7342*	800 College Court New Bern	28562				CC	PBL	12	12	17	20	17	17
004	Durham Tech Comm College Dr Louise J Gooche, Director *Chair's #: (919) 686-3673*	1637 Lawson St Durham	27703				TCH	PBL	12	12	38	40	26	25
023	Fayetteville Tech Comm College Mrs Kathy T Weeks, Chair *Chair's #: (910) 678-8482*	PO Box 35236 Fayetteville	28303				CC	PBL	11	12	26	24	24	26

NORTH CAROLINA

- Continued

School Code	Name of School, Director of Program, and Phone Number	Street Address / City or Town and Zip Code	Footnotes	Type of Program	NLNAC Accreditation as of January 31, 1999	Administrative Control	Financial Support (principal source)	Number of Months in Program	Educational Requirements for Entering Adult Program	Enrollments as of October 15, 1998	Admissions Aug. 1, 1997 - July 31, 1998	Graduations Aug. 1, 1997 - July 31, 1998	Fall Admissions Aug. 1, 1998 - Dec. 31, 1998
012	Forsyth Tech Comm College Mrs Carolyn Rajacich, Asst Dean *Chair's #: (336) 723-0371 Ext 7416*	2100 Silas Creek Pkwy Winston-Salem 27103				CC	PBL			Publication withheld			
060	Gaston College-LincolnCenter Mrs Beverly Davis, Chair *Chair's #: (704) 922-6400*	511 South Aspen St Lincolnton 28092				CC	PBL	12	12	19	32	23	19
055	Isothermal Comm College Ms Debbie Sain Rogers, Director *Chair's #: (828) 286-3636 Ext 254*	PO Box 804 Spindale 28160				CC	PBL	12	12	24	24	24	24
005	James Sprunt Comm Coll Mrs Rhonda B Ferrell, Chair *Chair's #: (910) 296-2450*	PO Box 398 Kenansville 28349				CC	PBL	12	12	19	20	19	0
056	Lenoir Comm College Mrs Alexis Welch, Dean *Chair's #: (252) 527-6223 Ext 801*	PO Box 188 Kinston 28502				CC	PBL	12	12	16	20	11	20
062	McDowell Tech Comm Coll Ms Shirley Garcia, Dir *Chair's #: (828) 652-6021 Ext 711*	Rt #1, Box 170 Marion 28752				CC	PBL			20	20	16	20
049	Montgomery Comm College Mrs Deborah B Morton, Director *Chair's #: (910) 576-6222 Ext 205*	PO Box 787 Troy 27371				TCH	PBL	12	12	28	30	22	30
070	Rockingham Comm College Mrs Cathy Franklin-Griffin, Dean *Chair's #: (336) 342-4261 Ext 248*	PO Box 38 Wentworth 27375				CC	PBL			25	25	20	27
042	Sampson Comm Coll Mrs Mary Brown, Chair *Chair's #: (910) 592-8081 Ext 6510*	PO 318 Clinton 28329				CC	PBL	12	12	20	20	13	20
058	Sandhills Comm College-Nsg Dept Ms Star Mitchell, Coord *Chair's #: (910) 692-6185 Ext 606*	2200 Airport Rd Pinehurst 28374				CC	PBL			Publication withheld			
043	Southeastern Comm College Mrs Peggy Blackmon, Dean *Chair's #: (910) 642-7141 Ext 0240*	PO Box 151 Whiteville 28472				CC	PBL	12	12	21	25	19	25
006	Surry Comm Coll Ms Sharon S Kallam, Chair *Chair's #: (336) 386-8121 Ext 227*	PO Box 304 Dobson 27017				CC	PBL	12	12	29	30	23	30
052	Vance-Granville Comm College Mrs Beth Cusatis Phillips, Dir *Chair's #: (252) 492-2061 Ext 222*	PO Box 917 Henderson 27536	7			CC	PBL			Data reported w/AD prog			

Explanation of footnotes on page x

School Code	Name of School, Director of Program, and Phone Number	Street Address, City or Town and Zip Code		Footnotes	Type of Program	NLNAC Accreditation as of January 31, 1999	Administrative Control	Financial Support (principal source)	Number of Months in Program	Educational Requirements for Entering Adult Program	Enrollments as of October 15, 1998	Admissions Aug. 1, 1997 - July 31, 1998	Graduations Aug. 1, 1997 - July 31, 1998	Fall Admissions Aug. 1, 1998 - Dec. 31, 1998
	NORTH CAROLINA													
	- Continued													
007	Wayne Comm College Dr Cynthia B Archie, Dept Head *Chair's #: (919) 735-5151 Ext 297*	Box 8002 Goldsboro	27533				CC	PBL	12	12	19	18	10	19
	NORTH DAKOTA													
	6 Programs in 6 Schools													
007	Dickinson State Univ Dr Eileen Hubsky, Interim Chair *Chair's #: (701) 483-2131*	291 Campus Dr Dickinson	58601	7		A	CC	PBL			Data reported w/AD prog			
005	Fort Berthold Comm Coll Mrs Brenda Caranicas, Director *Chair's #: (701) 627-4738 Ext 254*	PO Box 490 New Town	58763				CC	PBL			43	33	10	34
004	North Dakota State College of Science Mrs Marlys Baumann, Chair *Chair's #: (701) 671-2967 Ext 2968*	800 6th N Wahpeton	58075			A	CC	PBL	18	12	105	53	62	30
900	Northwest Technical Coll Ms Mary Wiersma, Director *Chair's #: (218) 773-4556*	Highway 220 W East Grand Forks	56721				TCH	PBL			Also reports in MN			
009	United Tribes Tech College Dr Kathryn Zimmer, Director *Chair's #: (701) 255-3285 Ext 265*	3315 University Dr Bismarck	58504			A	CC	PVT	17	12	54	40	17	40
012	Univ of North Dakota-Williston Ms Linda Tharp, Chair *Chair's #: (701) 774-4290*	1410 Univ Ave Box 1326 Williston	58802				CC	PBL			Publication withheld			
	OHIO													
	45 Programs in 40 Schools													
001	Akron Sch of Practical Nursing Mrs Marilyn Barkley, Dir *Chair's #: (330) 761-3255*	619 Sumner St Akron	44311			A	SEC	PBL	11	12	56	60	53	57
015	Apollo Sch of PN Miss Ruth Speakman, Coord *Chair's #: (419) 998-2975*	3325 Shawnee Rd Lima	45806				SEC	PBL	0	12	30	35	29	31
026	Belmont Tech College-Sch of PN Mrs Rebecca Kurtz, Asst Dean *Chair's #: (740) 695-9500 Ext 1024*	120 Fox-Shannon Pl St Clairsville	43950				TCH	PBL	12	12	34	32	32	34
021	Butler Co Program of PN Ed Mrs Joyce Harris, Dir *Chair's #: (513) 868-6300 Ext 4203*	3603 Hamilton-Middletown Hamilton	45011				TCH	PBL	10	12	94	106	54	69
028	Central Ohio Tech Coll Ms Tamar Gilson, Chair *Chair's #: (740) 366-9285*	1179 Univerity Dr Newark	4305	2			TCH	PBL	12	12	9	0	0	9

School Code	Name of School, Director of Program, and Phone Number	Street Address / City or Town and Zip Code	Footnotes	Type of Program	NLNAC Accreditation as of January 31, 1999	Administrative Control	Financial Support (principal source)	Number of Months in Program	Educational Requirements for Entering Adult Program	Enrollments as of October 15, 1998	Admissions Aug. 1, 1997 - July 31, 1998	Graduations Aug. 1, 1997 - July 31, 1998	Fall Admissions Aug. 1, 1998 - Dec. 31, 1998
	OHIO												
	- Continued												
004	Central Sch of Practical Nursing, Inc Ms Nancy Giesser, Dir Chair's #: (216) 391-8434	4600 Carnegie Ave Cleveland 44103			A	IND	PVT	12	12	60	68	47	45
010	Choffin Sch of Practical Nursing Mrs Janet M Carpenter, Supv Chair's #: (330) 744-8722	200 East Wood St Youngstown 44503			A	TCH	PBL	10	12	55	57	40	56
002	Cincinnati Public Sch of PN Ms Roberta Russo, Director Chair's #: (513) 977-8081	425 Ezzard Charles Dr Cincinnati 45203				SEC	PBL	12	10	96	90	55	30
033	Clark State Comm College Mrs Carolyn Swanger, Dean Chair's #: (937) 328-6060	570 E Leffel Ln Box 570 Springfield 45501				TCH	PBL			Publication withheld			
058	Collins Career Center Mrs Wanda Huffman, Interim Dir Chair's #: (740) 867-6641 Ext 414	11627 St RT 243 Chesapeake 45619				TCH	PBL	11	12	32	42	28	38
012	Columbus Pub Schools - Sch of PN Ms Donna Thomas, Coord Chair's #: (614) 365-5241	100 Arcadia Ave Rm-300 W Columbus 43202				SEC	PBL			Publication withheld			
009	Cuyahoga Comm College--PN Prog Mrs Janice Melnick, Manager Chair's #: (216) 987-2276	4250 Richmond Rd Cleveland 44122	7			CC	PBL	10		24	38	26	26
019	EHOVE Sch of PN Miss Deborah Toth, Dir Chair's #: (419) 499-4663 Ext 284	316 West Mason Rd Milan 44846	2			TCH	PBL	12	12	43	36	25	44
014	Great Oaks Sch of PN Scarlet Oaks Care Mrs Lina Nichols, Dir Chair's #: (513) 771-8810 Ext 429	3254 E Kemper Rd Cincinnati 45241			A	TCH	PBL	11	12	117	91	56	77
017	Hannah E Mullins Sch of Practical Nsg Mrs Beverly Henderson, Dir Chair's #: (330) 332-8940	1200 E 6 th Salem 44460			A	TCH	PBL	11	12	49	57	27	31
040	Hocking Tech College Nsg Career Ladd Ms Molly Weiland, Dean Chair's #: (740) 753-3591 Ext 2215	3301 Hocking Pkwy Nelsonville 45764			A	TCH	PBL			220	260	158	60
047	Jefferson Comm Coll Miss Kathleen F Keenan, Director Chair's #: (740) 264-5591	4000 Sunset Blvd Steubenville 43952				TCH	PBL			Publication withheld			
055	Knoedler Sch of PN Ed Mrs Dawn Bleau, Dir Chair's #: (440) 576-6015 Ext 201	1565 Rt 167 Jefferson 44047				TCH	PBL	11	12	44	45	41	45

Explanation of footnotes on page x

School Code	Name of School, Director of Program, and Phone Number	Street Address / City or Town and Zip Code	Footnotes	Type of Program	NLNAC Accreditation as of January 31, 1999	Administrative Control	Financial Support (principal source)	Number of Months in Program	Educational Requirements for Entering Adult Program	Enrollments as of October 15, 1998	Admissions Aug. 1, 1997 - July 31, 1998	Graduations Aug. 1, 1997 - July 31, 1998	Fall Admissions Aug. 1, 1998 - Dec. 31, 1998
	OHIO **- Continued**												
053	Knox Co Career Center Mrs Waynette Bridwell, Coord *Chair's #: (740) 397-5820 Ext 269*	306 Martinsburg Rd Mt Vernon 43050				TCH	PBL	11	12	30	33	24	31
025	Lima Tech College Dr Lois Deleruyelle, Chair *Chair's #: (419) 995-8218*	4240 Campus Dr Lima 45804	2			CC	PBL			Publication withheld			
041	Lorain County Comm College PN Progr Mr Robert A Schloss, Dir *Chair's #: (440) 366-4016*	1005 N Abbe Rd Elyria 44035			A	CC	PBL	11	12	68	0	51	68
006	Marymount Sch of Practical Nursing Ms Suzan Leonard, Dir *Chair's #: (216) 587-8160 Ext 2439*	12300 McCracken Rd Garfield Hts 44125			A	HSP	PVT	12	12	18	27	24	36
003	Miami Valley Career Tech Ms Frances Childers, Dir *Chair's #: (937) 854-6370*	6800 Hoke Rd Clayton 45315				TCH	PBL			65	80	55	0
039	Mid-East OH Voc Sch Syst Adult&Cont Mrs Cathy Learn, Coord *Chair's #: (740) 455-3111 Ext 147*	400 Richards Rd Zanesville 43701				TCH	PBL	11	12	46	54	43	51
044	Muskingum Perry Career Center Mrs Cathy Learn, Coord *Chair's #: (740) 455-3111 Ext 147*	400 Richards Rd Zanesville 43701				TCH	PBL			0	0	0	0
			HS			TCH	PBL	18		35	22	15	0
052	North Central Tech College Ms Carol Lepley, Director *Chair's #: (419) 755-4823*	2441 Kenwood Circle Box 698 Mansfield 44901				CC	PBL	12	12	55	63	63	32
048	Northwest St Comm College Mrs Karen Short, Coord *Chair's #: (419) 267-5511 Ext 253*	22 600 St Rt 34 Archbold 43502				CC	PBL	12	12	24	35	38	27
061	Ohio Hi-Point Joint Voc Sch of PN Ms Darlene C Chiles, Supv *Chair's #: (937) 599-6275 Ext 210*	2280 State Rt 540 Bellefontaine 43311				TCH	PBL	12	12	31	36	21	36
030	Parma Sch of PN Mrs Myrna George, Supv *Chair's #: (440) 885-2364*	6726 Ridge Rd Parma 44129				SEC	PBL			Publication withheld			
065	Pickaway-Ross Co JVSD Mrs Mary Van Sickle, Coord *Chair's #: (740) 773-6873*	Bldg 4 17273 St Rd 104 Chillicothe 45601			A	TCH	PBL	10	12	29	34	26	34
037	PN Program of Canton City Schs Mrs Judy Stauder, Coord *Chair's #: (330) 453-3271*	1253 Third St SE Canton 44707			A	SEC	PBL	12	12	58	86	46	86

Explanation of footnotes on page x

School Code	Name of School, Director of Program, and Phone Number	Street Address, City or Town and Zip Code		Footnotes	Type of Program	NLNAC Accreditation as of January 31, 1999	Administrative Control	Financial Support (principal source)	Number of Months in Program	Educational Requirements for Entering Adult Program	Enrollments as of October 15, 1998	Admissions Aug. 1, 1997 - July 31, 1998	Graduations Aug. 1, 1997 - July 31, 1998	Fall Admissions Aug. 1, 1998 - Dec. 31, 1998
	OHIO													
	- Continued													
051	PN Program of Scioto Co JVS Ms Brenda J Horr, Director Chair's #: (614) 259-5522	PO Box 766 Lucasville	45648				TCH	PBL			Publication withheld			
050	PN Sch-Buckeye Hills Career Ctr Mrs Phyllis Pope-Brown, Coord Chair's #: (614) 245-5334 Ext 206	PO Box 157 351 Buckeye Hills Rio Grande	45674				TCH	PBL			Publication withheld			
034	Portage Lakes Car Ctr W Howard Nicol Mrs Mary Ann Cosgarea, Coord Chair's #: (330) 896-8105	4401 Shriver Rd PO Box 248 Green	44232				TCH	PBL	11	12	34	34	29	34
060	Southern State Comm College Mrs Jo Carol Laymon, Director Chair's #: (937) 393-3431 Ext 2640	200 Hobart Dr Hillsboro	45133				CC	PBL	11	12	31	41	22	0
020	The Stautzenberger Coll Ms Jane Ridge, Coord Chair's #: (419) 423-2211	1637 Tiffine Ave Findlay	45840	2			TCH	PVT	17	12	58	113	59	63
008	Toledo Sch of PN-Woodward Ms Veronica Backman, Coord Chair's #: (419) 244-8301	1602 Washington St Toledo	43624				SEC	PBL			Publication withheld			
016	Tri-Rivers Sch of PN Dr Judith R Higel, Manager Chair's #: (740) 389-4681 Ext 125	2222 Marion Mt Gilead Rd Marion	43302				TCH	PBL	10	12	34	92	40	44
067	Trumbull Co Joint Voc Sch Mrs Linda Reader, Coord Chair's #: (330) 847-0503 Ext 326	528 Education Highway Warren	44483		HS		TCH TCH	PBL PBL	18	12	14 20	7 12	3 4	6 13
054	Upper Valley JVS Sch of PN Ms Doris Luckett, Admin Chair's #: (937) 778-1980 Ext 253	8811 Career Dr Piqua	45356				TCH	PBL	17	12	50	48	27	21
023	Washington State Comm College Mrs Ann Stewart, Dir Chair's #: (740) 374-8716 Ext 671	710 Colegate Dr Marietta	45750				CC	PBL			Publication withheld			
046	Wayne Adult Sch of PN (2 Progs) Mrs Kathy Sommers, Coord Chair's #: (330) 669-2134 Ext 208	518 W Prospect St Smithville	44677		HS		TCH TCH	PBL PBL	12 18	12 12	39 32	40 20	28 0	40 20
036	Willoughby-Eastlk Sch of PN (2 Progs) Mrs Barbara Sesler, Dir Chair's #: (440) 946-7085 Ext 1	25 Public Square Willoughby	44094				SEC	PBL			26	26	21	26

Explanation of footnotes on page x

School Code	Name of School, Director of Program, and Phone Number	Street Address	City or Town and Zip Code	Footnotes	Type of Program	NLNAC Accreditation as of January 31, 1999	Administrative Control	Financial Support (principal source)	Number of Months in Program	Educational Requirements for Entering Adult Program	Enrollments as of October 15, 1998	Admissions Aug. 1, 1997 - July 31, 1998	Graduations Aug. 1, 1997 - July 31, 1998	Fall Admissions Aug. 1, 1998 - Dec. 31, 1998
	OKLAHOMA													
	31 Programs in 31 Schools													
022	Autry Technology Center, Mrs Barbara Simmons, Coord, *Chair's #: (580) 242-2750 Ext 163*	1201 W Willow	Enid 73073			A	TCH	PBL			Publication withheld			
035	Caddo-Kiowa Area Voc-Tech Sch Dist 2, Ms Marquita Lindsey, Coord, *Chair's #: (405) 643-5511 Ext 263*	PO Box 90	Ft Cobb 73015			A	TCH	PBL	15	12	24	40	28	14
027	Canadian Valley Area AVTS-Dist 6, Mrs Angela M Siegrist, Coordinator, *Chair's #: (405) 422-2353*	6505 E Hwy 66	El Reno 73036			A	TCH	PBL	18	10	24	24	24	24
021	Canadian Valley AVTS, Mrs Rhonda Reherman, Director, *Chair's #: (405) 224-7220 Ext 792*	1401 Michigan Ave	Chichasha 73018			A	TCH	PBL	24	12	36	32	20	0
024	Central OK Area Voc-Tech Sch Dist 3, Ms Carla J Brittenham, Coord, *Chair's #: (918) 352-2551 Ext 288*	3 C T Circle	Drumright 74030			A	TCH	PBL	12	12	40	49	40	25
076	Chisholm Trail Area Voc-Tech Sch, Mrs Carla Maloy, Coord, *Chair's #: (405) 729-8324*	Rt 1 Box 60	Omega 73764			A	TCH	PBL	12	12	12	14	12	13
063	Demarge College, Ms Sandi White, Dir, *Chair's #: (405) 692-2900 Ext 23*	3608 H W 58th St	Oklahoma City 73142				TCH	PVT	18	12	95	96	33	56
042	Francis Tuttle Voc-Tech Ctr PN Prog, Mrs Linda Dawkins, Coord, *Chair's #: (405) 717-4128*	12777 N Rockwell	Oklahoma City 73142			A	TCH	PBL	11	12	33	31	22	26
026	Gordon Cooper Technology Center, Mrs Lisa Morlan, Coord, *Chair's #: (405) 273-7493 Ext 291*	One John C Bruton Blvd	Shawnee 74801				TCH	PBL	11	12	24	26	22	25
010	GPAVTS Dist 9, Ms LaDonna Meyer, Dir, *Chair's #: (580) 250-5595*	4500 W Lee Blvd	Lawton 73505			A	TCH	PBL	12	12	30	60	60	30
900	Green Country AVTS, Ms Molly Parker, Director, *Chair's #: (918) 758-0840*	PO Box 1217	Okmulgee 74047				TCH	PBL	12	12	15	20	18	0
012	High Plains AVTS Sch of PN, Ms Sue Mitchell, Dir, *Chair's #: (580) 571-6159*	3921 34th St	Woodward 73801				TCH	PBL	12	12	23	17	17	24
011	Indian Captl Voc-Tech Sch (4 Campus, Mrs Debra A Bartel, Coord, *Chair's #: (918) 775-9119 Ext 108*	H C 61 Box 12	Sallisaw 74955			A	TCH	PBL	15	12	85	90	64	72

School Code	Name of School, Director of Program, and Phone Number	Street Address	City or Town and Zip Code	Footnotes	Type of Program	NLNAC Accreditation as of January 31, 1999	Administrative Control	Financial Support (principal source)	Number of Months in Program	Educational Requirements for Entering Adult Program	Enrollments as of October 15, 1998	Admissions Aug. 1, 1997 - July 31, 1998	Graduations Aug. 1, 1997 - July 31, 1998	Fall Admissions Aug. 1, 1998 - Dec. 31, 1998
	OKLAHOMA													
	- Continued													
039	Kiamichi Area Voc-Tech (8 Campuses) Mrs Sherry Payne Burke, Director *Chair's #: (918) 567-2264 Ext 24*	Rt 2 Box 1800	Talihina 74571			A	TCH	PBL	12	12	155	144	132	156
032	Meridian Technology Center Mrs Dolores Cotton, Coord *Chair's #: (405) 377-3333 Ext 324*	1312 S Sangre Rd	Stillwater 74074			A	TCH	PBL	12	12	32	33	28	27
004	Metro Area Voc Technical School Mrs Deborah Kamphaus, Coord *Chair's #: (405) 424-8324 Ext 610*	1720 Springlake Dr	Oklahoma City 73111			A	TCH	PBL	15	12	39	42	22	44
030	Mid-America Area Voc-Tech Sch Dist 8 Mrs Gina Doyle, Coord *Chair's #: (405) 449-3391 Ext 265*	PO Box H	Wayne 73095			A	TCH	PBL	11	12	29	30	25	29
017	Mid-Del Lewis Eubanks AVTS Mrs Vivian Bingman, Dir *Chair's #: (405) 739-1713*	1621 Maple Dr	Midwest City 73110	HSE		A A	TCH TCH	PBL PBL	16 16	11	13 13	16 21	13 1	15 14
020	Moore-Norman Technology Center Ms Naomi R Jones, Asst Dir *Chair's #: (405) 364-5763 Ext 349*	4701 12th Ave NW	Norman 73069			A	TCH	PBL	10	12	48	48	45	50
029	Northeast Area Voc-Tech Sch (3 Campu Ms Teresa Fraizer, Coord *Chair's #: (918) 257-8324 Ext 49*	PO Box 487	Pryor 74362			A	TCH	PBL	11	12	62	63	45	66
031	Pioneer Area Voc-Tech Sch Dist 13 Mrs Mary E Frantz, Coord *Chair's #: (580) 762-8336 Ext 251*	2101 N Ash	Ponca City 74601				GOV	PBL	11	12	22	26	26	24
001	Platt College (2 campuses) Ms Kay Haywood, Dir *Chair's #: (405) 946-7799 Ext 23*	309 S Ann Arbor Ave	Oklahoma City 73128				TCH	PVT			Publication withheld			
008	Pontotoc Technology Center Mrs Penny Stone, Dir *Chair's #: (580) 310-2258*	601 W 33rd	Ada 74820				TCH	PBL	11	12	24	30	24	31
033	Red River Area V-T Sch Dist 19 Mrs Earlene K Werner, Dir *Chair's #: (580) 255-2903 Ext 237*	PO Box 1807	Duncan 73533			A	TCH	PBL	12	12	26	26	20	26
023	School of Tech Training Ms Verna Reid, Director *Chair's #: (405) 355-4416*	112 S W 11th St	Lawton 73501				TCH	PVT			46	39	28	17
019	Southern Oklahoma Area Voc-Tech Ctr Ms Sylvia Diggs, Coord *Chair's #: (580) 223-2070*	Rt 1 Box 14M	Ardmore 73401				TCH	PBL			Publication withheld			

Explanation of footnotes on page x

School Code	Name of School, Director of Program, and Phone Number	Street Address, City or Town and Zip Code		Footnotes	Type of Program	NLNAC Accreditation as of January 31, 1999	Administrative Control	Financial Support (principal source)	Number of Months in Program	Educational Requirements for Entering Adult Program	Enrollments as of October 15, 1998	Admissions Aug. 1, 1997 - July 31, 1998	Graduations Aug. 1, 1997 - July 31, 1998	Fall Admissions Aug. 1, 1998 - Dec. 31, 1998
	OKLAHOMA													
	- Continued													
043	Southwest OK Sch PN Mrs Elva Pruitt, Dir *Chair's #: (580) 477-2250 Ext 257*	1121 North Spurgeon Altus	73521					TCH	PBL	12	12	26	29	23	0
005	Tri-Co Area Voc-Tech Sch Dist 1 Mrs Ruth Howell, Dir *Chair's #: (918) 331-3223*	6101 Nowata Rd Bartlesville	74006				A	TCH	PBL	0	12	28	33	22	0
009	Tulsa Technology Center Ms Rita Hejtmanick, Coord *Chair's #: (918) 828-1043*	3420 S Memorial Dr Tulsa	74145				A	TCH	PBL			Publication withheld			
045	Wes Watkins Technology Center Ms Linda Sanford Campbell, Coord *Chair's #: (405) 452-5500 Ext 277*	Route 2 Box 159-1 Wetumka	74883					TCH	PBL	12	12	28	21	20	14
028	Western Technology Center Mrs Marianne Doss, Coord *Chair's #: (580) 562-3181 Ext 2264*	621 Sooner Dr PO Box 1469 Burns Flat	73624				A	TCH	PBL	12	12	34	36	31	1
	OREGON													
	11 Programs in 11 Schools													
009	Blue Mountain Comm College PN Prog Mrs Elizabeth Sullivan, Chair *Chair's #: (541) 278-5879*	PO Box 100 Pendleton	97801		7			CC	PBL			Data reported w/AD prog			
004	Central Oregon Comm College PN Prog Mr Doug McCready, Dir *Chair's #: (541) 383-7546*	2600 NW College Way Bend	97701		7			CC	PBL			Data reported w/AD prog			
007	Chemeketa Comm College Dr Doris Williams, Dir *Chair's #: (503) 399-5058*	4000 Lancaster Dr, NE Salem	97309		7			CC	PBL			Data repoorted w/AD prog			
016	Clackamas Comm College PN Prog Mrs Arlene Jurgens, Chair *Chair's #: (503) 657-6958 Ext 2428*	19600 S Molalla Ave Oregon City	97045		7			CC	PBL			Data reported w/AD prog			
017	Clatsop Comm College Ms Karen M Burke, Dir *Chair's #: (503) 338-2496*	1653 Jerome Ave Astoria	97103		7			CC	PBL			Data reported w/AD prog			
006	Lane Comm College PN Prog Ms Joyce Godels, Chair *Chair's #: (503) 747-4501 Ext 2619*	4000 E 30th Ave Eugene	97405		7			CC	PBL			Data reported w/AD Prog			
015	Mt Hood Comm College PN Prog P Gubrud and M Westphal, Co Dirs *Chair's #: (503) 667-7404*	26000 SE Stark Gresham	97030		7			CC	PBL			Data reported w/AD prog			

School Code	Name of School, Director of Program, and Phone Number	Street Address / City or Town and Zip Code		Footnotes	Type of Program	NLNAC Accreditation as of January 31, 1999	Administrative Control	Financial Support (principal source)	Number of Months in Program	Educational Requirements for Entering Adult Program	Enrollments as of October 15, 1998	Admissions Aug. 1, 1997 - July 31, 1998	Graduations Aug. 1, 1997 - July 31, 1998	Fall Admissions Aug. 1, 1998 - Dec. 31, 1998
	OREGON													
	- Continued													
010	Rogue Comm College Mrs Linda Wagner, Director *Chair's #: (541) 471-3500 Ext 268*	3345 Redwood Hwy Grants Pass	97527	7			CC	PBL			Data reported w/AD prog			
012	SW Oregon Comm College PN Sch Ms Kristen Crusoe, Dir *Chair's #: (503) 888-7343*	1988 Newmark Coos Bay	97420	7			CC	PBL			Data reported w/AD Prog			
013	Treasure Valley Comm College PN Prog Mrs Maureen McDonough, Director *Chair's #: (541) 889-6493 Ext 345*	650 College Blvd Ontario	97914				CC	PBL	9	12	23	24	20	26
014	Umpqua Comm College PN Prog Mr Duane D Alexenko, Dir *Chair's #: (541) 440-4613*	PO Box 967 Roseburg	97470	7			CC	PBL			Data reported w/AD prog			
	PENNSYLVANIA													
	47 Programs in 47 Schools													
055	Career Tech Center of Lakawanna Co Mrs Sallie Noto, Supv *Chair's #: (717) 346-8728*	3201 Rockwell Ave Scranton	18508				A	TCH	PBL	12	12	53	64	28	41
031	Alvernia School-St Francis Med Center Miss Lois McKinley, Dir *Chair's #: (412) 622-4496*	400 45th St Pittsburgh	15201				A	HSP	PVT	12	12	16	25	13	0
021	Bucks County Technical School Ms Mendy Blumberg, Coordinator *Chair's #: (215) 949-1700 Ext 32*	610 Wistar Rd Fairless Hills	19030	2			A	TCH	PBL	12	12	29	34	24	33
013	Center for Arts & Technology Ms Patty Knecht, Dir *Chair's #: (610) 384-1585 Ext 216*	1635 E Lincoln Hwy Coatesville	19320				A	TCH	PBL			62	51	42	58
018	Central PA Inst of Science and Tech Mrs Ellouise Garver, Coord *Chair's #: (814) 359-2582 Ext 265*	540 N Harrison Rd Pleasant Gap	16823				A	TCH	PBL	12	12	16	16	16	0
057	Central Susquehanna Career Center Ms Kay Yannaccone, Dir *Chair's #: (717) 437-3176*	DeLong Building Box 140 Washingtonville	17884				A	IND	PBL	12	12	59	62	69	36
074	Clarion Co Area Voc-Tech School Mrs Barbara Barger, Coord *Chair's #: (814) 226-5857*	1976 Career Way Shippenville	16254				A	TCH	PBL	12	12	39	42	32	12
068	Clearfield Co Area Voc Tech School Ms Elsie Reichard, Coord *Chair's #: (814) 765-4047*	RR #1 Box 5 Clearfield	16830				A	TCH	PBL	12	12	32	33	31	20

Explanation of footnotes on page x

School Code	Name of School, Director of Program, and Phone Number	Street Address / City or Town and Zip Code		Footnotes	Type of Program	NLNAC Accreditation as of January 31, 1998	Administrative Control	Financial Support (principal source)	Number of Months in Program	Educational Requirements for Entering Adult Program	Enrollments as of October 15, 1998	Admissions Aug. 1, 1997 - July 31, 1998	Graduations Aug. 1, 1997 - July 31, 1998	Fall Admissions Aug. 1, 1998 - Dec. 31, 1998
	PENNSYLVANIA													
	- Continued													
051	Comm College of Beaver County Mrs Linda Gallagher, Dir *Chair's #: (724) 775-8561 Ext 200*	1 Campus Dr Monaca	15061	7			CC	PBL			Data reported w/AD Prog			
064	Crawford County Area Voc Tech School Dr Carol Vogt, Dir *Chair's #: (814) 724-6028*	860 Thurston Rd Meadville	16335		A		TCH	PBL	12	12	21	21	17	22
002	Delaware Co Area Voc-Tech Sch Mrs Catherine Coakley, Coord *Chair's #: (610) 583-2934 Ext 221*	Delmar Dr & Henderson Blvd Folcroft	19032		A		TCH	PBL	12	12	63	68	39	39
044	Eastern Center for Arts and Technology Mrs Barbara Gravel, Supervisor *Chair's #: (215) 784-4805*	3075 Terwood Rd Willow Grove	19090		A		TCH	PBL	12	12	52	42	31	43
043	Fayette Co Area Voc Tech School Mrs Marilyn Tyhonas, Coord *Chair's #: (724) 437-2724*	RD #2, Box 122A Uniontown	15401		A		TCH	PBL	12	12	48	55	49	18
900	Forbes Rd East Area Voc Tech School Mrs Edna Litwiller, Coord *Chair's #: (412) 373-8100 Ext 232*	607 Beatty Rd Monroeville	15146				TCH	PBL	12	12	17	21	16	12
019	Franklin Co Career and Tech Center Mrs Mary E Butts, Admin *Chair's #: (717) 263-5667*	2463 Loop Rd Chambersburg	17201		A		TCH	PBL	12	12	65	75	65	38
032	Greater Altoona Career Tech Center Mrs Margaret O'Brien, Coord *Chair's #: (814) 946-8490*	1500 4th Ave Altoona	16602				TCH	PBL	12	12	40	37	24	40
005	Greater Johnstown Area Voc Tech Scho Mrs Bonnie Ford Boroski, Coord *Chair's #: (814) 269-4393 Ext 2217*	445 Schoolhouse Rd Johnstown	15904		A		TCH	PVT	12	12	45	53	33	35
067	Greene County Area Voc Tech School Mrs Patsy Trump, Coord *Chair's #: (724) 627-3106 Ext 208*	60 Zimmerman Dr Waynesburg	15370		A		TCH	PBL	12	12	20	18	25	26
041	Hanover Public School Dist Mrs Shirley LeDane, Coord *Chair's #: (717) 637-2111 Ext 0204*	403 Moul Ave Hanover	17331		A		SEC	PVT	12	12	27	32	29	0
084	Harrisburg Area Comm College Mr Ronald Rebuck, Coord *Chair's #: (717) 780-2344*	One HACC Dr Harrisburg	17110		A		CC	PBL	12	12	30	40	28	40
066	Hazleton Area Voc Tech School Ms Bernice Platek, Coord *Chair's #: (570) 459-3178*	1451 West 23rd St Hazleton	18201		A		TCH	PVT	12	12	27	28	27	0

School Code	Name of School, Director of Program, and Phone Number	Street Address / City or Town and Zip Code		Footnotes	Type of Program	NLNAC Accreditation as of January 31, 1999	Administrative Control	Financial Support (principal source)	Number of Months in Program	Educational Requirements for Entering Adult Program	Enrollments as of October 15, 1998	Admissions Aug. 1, 1997 - July 31, 1998	Graduations Aug. 1, 1997 - July 31, 1998	Fall Admissions Aug. 1, 1998 - Dec. 31, 1998
062	Indiana Co Area Voc-Tech School Mrs Sharon Powell Laney, Coord *Chair's #: (724) 349-6700 Ext 121*	441 Hamill Rd Indiana	15701			A	TCH	PBL	12	12	52	48	33	39
053	Jefferson Co-Dubois Area Voc Tech Sch Mrs Marion Monahan, Coord *Chair's #: (814) 653-8265*	100 Jeff Tech Dr Reynoldsville	15851	2		A	TCH	PBL	12	12	18	24	16	0
065	Juniata-Mifflin Co Area Voc Tech Sch Ms Marcia Dedmon, Coord *Chair's #: (717) 248-3933*	700 Pittt St Lewistown	17044			A	TCH	PBL	12	12	38	53	39	15
023	Lancaster Co Career and Tech Center Ms Wanda McGarvey, Coord *Chair's #: (717) 464-7050 Ext 7063*	1730 Hans-Herr Dr Box 527 Willow Street	17584			A	TCH	PBL	12	12	97	99	81	25
054	Lawrence County Area Voc-Tech Schoo Mrs Marlene Stoddard, Coord *Chair's #: (724) 654-2810*	750 Phelps Way New Castle	16101	2		A	TCH	PBL	12	12	12	31	20	0
024	Lebanon Co Area Voc-Tech School Mrs Lynda Maurer, Supv *Chair's #: (717) 273-4401*	833 Metro Dr Lebanon	17042			A	TCH	PBL	12	12	40	49	40	44
016	Lehigh Carbon Comm College Mrs Mary Karen Shoff, Coord *Chair's #: (610) 799-1547*	4525 Education Park Dr Schnecksville	18078			A	CC	PBL	12	12	26	31	0	0
075	Lenape Area Voc-Tech School Ms Rebecca A Cappo, Coord *Chair's #: (724) 763-2608*	2215 Chaplin Ave Ford City	16226			A	TCH	PBL	12		73	80	60	29
063	Mercer County Area Voc Tech Sch Ms Jean Fobes, Coord *Chair's #: (724) 662-6730 Ext 26*	776 Greenville Rd Box 152 Mercer	16137				TCH	PBL		Publication withheld				
076	Monroe Co Area Voc-Tech School Ms Sheila M Carolan, Coord *Chair's #: (717) 629-6563*	PO Box 66 Laurel Lake Dr Bartonsville	18321			A	TCH	PBL	12	12	28	27	32	29
071	Northampton Comm Coll Ms Aurora Weaver, Dir *Chair's #: (610) 861-5376*	3835 Green Pond Rd Bethlehem	18020			A	CC	PBL		Data reported w/AD prog				
080	Northern Tier Career Center Mrs Dorothy M Bennett, Coord *Chair's #: (717) 265-8113 Ext 25*	RR #1 Box 157A Towanda	18848			A	TCH	PBL	12	12	19	24	13	20
036	PA College of Technology Ms Pamela Starcher, Dir *Chair's #: (570) 327-4525*	One College Ave Williamsport	17701				COL	PBL	16	12	16	13	0	10

Explanation of footnotes on page x

School Code	Name of School, Director of Program, and Phone Number	Street Address, City or Town and Zip Code	Footnotes	Type of Program	NLNAC Accreditation as of January 31, 1999	Administrative Control	Financial Support (principal source)	Number of Months in Program	Educational Requirements for Entering Adult Program	Enrollments as of October 15, 1998	Admissions Aug. 1, 1997 - July 31, 1998	Graduations Aug. 1, 1997 - July 31, 1998	Fall Admissions Aug. 1, 1998 - Dec. 31, 1998
	PENNSYLVANIA												
	- Continued												
087	Parkway West Voc-Tech Sch Mrs Cindy Fickley, Coord *Chair's #: (412) 923-1772 Ext 140*	7101 Steubenville Pike Oakdale 15071			A	TCH	PBL	12	12	16	12	10	19
001	Pittsburgh Public Schs-Connelley Tech Dr Patricia Mashburn, Coord *Chair's #: (412) 338-3720*	1501 Bedford Ave Pittsburgh 15219				TCH	PBL	12	12	44	40	52	27
015	Reading Area Comm College Mrs Elissa S Sauer, Asst Dean *Chair's #: (610) 372-4721 Ext 5420*	10 S Second St PO Box 1706 Reading 19603			A	CC	PBL	12	12	39	38	33	43
022	Sch District of the City of Erie Miss Sheila M Warner, Coord *Chair's #: (814) 868-3345*	2931 Harvard Rd Erie 16508			A	TCH	PBL	12	12	22	34	16	0
048	Schuylkill Training & Tech Center Ms Karen Runk, Dir *Chair's #: (717) 874-1034 Ext 4880*	101 Technology Dr Frackville 17931			A	TCH	PBL	12	12	53	62	47	0
049	Somerset County Tech Center Ms Sibyl McNelly, Coord *Chair's #: (814) 445-8522*	6022 Glades Pike Suite 180 Somerset 15501			A	TCH	PBL	12	12	29	29	25	17
038	Univ of PA-Presbysteriam Med Ctr Mrs Anna M Marshalick, Director *Chair's #: (215) 662-9164*	39th St and Market Sts Philadelphia 19104			A	HSP	PVT			Publication withheld			
042	Upper Bucks Co Area Voc-Tech School Mrs Rachel Swierzewski, Supv *Chair's #: (215) 795-2234 Ext 224*	3115 Ridge Rd Perkasie 18944			A	TCH	PBL	12	12	33	42	36	33
047	Venango Co Area Voc-Tech Sch Ms Sally Bowser, Coord *Chair's #: (814) 677-3097 Ext 207*	1 Voc-Tech Dr Oil City 16301			A	TCH	PVT	11	12	28	29	16	29
078	Western Area Career and Tech Center Mrs Nancy Lohr, Coord *Chair's #: (724) 746-2890 Ext 117*	688 Western Ave Canonsburg 15317			A	TCH	PBL	12	12	26	30	28	0
028	Westmoreland County Comm College Dr Patricia Milhalcin, Div Chair *Chair's #: (724) 925-4028*	Armbrust Rd Youngwood 15697	7			CC	PBL			Data reported w/AD prog			
026	Wilkes-Barre Area Voc Tech School Ms Mary M Cawley, Coord *Chair's #: (717) 822-6539*	Box 1699 Jumper Rd Wilkes-Barre 18705			A	TCH	PBL	12	12	69	59	47	25
037	York County Area Voc-Tech School Ms Barbara Garzon, Admin *Chair's #: (717) 741-0820 Ext 256*	2179 S Queen St York 17402			A	TCH	PBL	11	12	34	65	54	31

School Code	Name of School, Director of Program, and Phone Number	Street Address City or Town and Zip Code	Footnotes	Type of Program	NLNAC Accreditation as of January 31, 1999	Administrative Control	Financial Support (principal source)	Number of Months in Program	Educational Requirements for Entering Adult Program	Enrollments as of October 15, 1998	Admissions Aug. 1, 1997 - July 31, 1998	Graduations Aug. 1, 1997 - July 31, 1998	Fall Admissions Aug. 1, 1998 - Dec. 31, 1998
	PUERTO RICO												
	45 Programs in 45 Schools												
023	Antilles Sch of Tech Careers Inc Mrs Carmen Ramirez, President *Chair's #: (787) 764-7576 Ext 0030*	PO Box 1536 Hato Rey 00919			A	TCH	PVT	15	12	31	10	29	5
006	Antonio Luchetti Voc HS Ms Bedzaida Font, Coord *Chair's #: (787) 881-3443 Ext 30*	PO Box 601 Arecibo 00612				TCH	PBL			Publication withheld			
026	Area Voc & Tech School-C F Daniels Mr Pagan Roche, Dir *Chair's #: (787) 762-7272*	Calle Jose Severo Quinones Carolina 00630				TCH	PBL			Publication withheld			
083	Atenas College Ms Maria Hernandez, Dir *Chair's #: (787) 884-3838*	PO Box 30160 Suite 146 Manati 00674				CC	PBL			Publication withheld			
008	Bernardino Cordero Voc HS Mrs Basilia Quiles, Coord *Chair's #: (787) 842-7091 Ext 28*	Juan B Roman Ave Ponce 00731				TCH	PBL			Publication withheld			
062	Caribbean Educ & Training Corp Ms L Feliciano, Dir *Chair's #: (787) 250-1272*	America #411 Hato Rey 00919				TCH	PBL			Publication withheld			
032	Centro de Estudios Multidisciplinarios Miss Adriana Toledo, Dir *Chair's #: (787) 852-5505*	Calle 13 1206 Urb San Agustin Humacao 00661				TCH	PVT			Publication withheld			
001	Centro de Estudios Multidisciplinarios Miss Adriana Toledo, Dir *Chair's #: (787) 765-4210 Ext 130*	602 Barbosa Ave Rio Piedras 00917				TCH	PVT			Publication withheld			
024	Colegio Tecnico de PR Ms Magali Estronga, Dir *Chair's #: (787) 267-5413*	Box 3020 Yauco 00698				CC	PBL			Publication withheld			
047	D'Carmen Beauty & Tech Coll Ms Carmen Rodriguez, Dir *Chair's #: (787) 852-8655*	Box 38 Humacao 00791	6			CC	PVT			Publication withheld			
011	Dr Pedro Perea Voc HS Ms Gladys Hernandez, Director *Chair's #: (787) 833-0865*	PO Box 1330 Mayaguez 00681				TCH	PBL			Publication withheld			
009	Escuela Superior Vocacional Ms Melva A Gonzales, Director *Chair's #: (787) 890-2935*	PO Box 296 Ramey 00604				TCH	PBL			Publication withheld			
013	Escuela Tecnica Vocacional Mrs Rosa Vazquez, Dir *Chair's #: (787) 250-7502*	PO Box 150 Guayama 00654				TCH	PBL			Publication withheld			

Explanation of footnotes on page x

School Code	Name of School, Director of Program, and Phone Number	Street Address, City or Town and Zip Code	Footnotes	Type of Program	NLNAC Accreditation as of January 31, 1999	Administrative Control	Financial Support (principal source)	Number of Months in Program	Educational Requirements for Entering Adult Program	Enrollments as of October 15, 1998	Admissions Aug. 1, 1997 - July 31, 1998	Graduations Aug. 1, 1997 - July 31, 1998	Fall Admissions Aug. 1, 1998 - Dec. 31, 1998
	PUERTO RICO												
	- Continued												
004	Escuela Voc Metro Miguel Such Dr Teresa Brana-Ortega, Professor *Chair's #: (787 751-3780*	PO Box 21837 Upr Station Rio Piedras 00931				GOV	PBL			Publication withheld			
040	Instituto de Banca y Comercio Mrs Mercedes Burgos, Director *Chair's #: (787) 738-7144*	PO Box 372710 Cayey 00737				TCH	PVT			Publication withheld			
037	Instituto de Banca y Comercio Ms Vivian Marrero, Counselor *Chair's #: (787) 854-6709*	Ave Munoz Rivera #996 Rio Piedras 00925				TCH	PVT			Publication withheld			
044	Instituto Irma Valentin Ms Irma Valentin, President *Chair's #: (787) 894-1395*	Dr Cueto # 137 Utuado 00641	6			TCH	PBL			Publication withheld			
068	John Dewey College Ms Jeliza Feliciano, Dir *Chair's #: (787) 769-1515*	PO Box 19538 San Juan 00910				CC	PBL			Publication withheld			
022	Jose A Montanez Genaro Mrs Natividad Calderon, Professor *Chair's #: (787) 854-2250*	Carr 2 Km 47.3 PO Box 1091 Manati 00701				TCH	PBL			Publication withheld			
018	Jose N Gandara HS-Voc Prog Ms Nydia Perez Linares, Instructor *Chair's #: (787) 735-9072*	PO Box 1269 Aibonito 00609				SEC	PBL			Publication withheld			
016	Luis Munoz Rivera HS Mr Juan Reyes, Director *Chair's #: (787) 894-2666*	Box 70 Utuado 00761		HS		GOV GOV	PBL PBL	10 30	12 12	16 0	14 0	10 0	16 10
055	Metro College Ms Carmen Maldonado, Dean *Chair's #: (787) 754-7120 Ext 223*	Ponce De Leon # 1126 San Juan 00925				TCH	PBL			Publication withheld			
049	Metro College Ms E Torres, Coordinator *Chair's #: (787) 259-7272*	123 Calle Villa Ponce 00731				CC	PBL			Publication withheld			
085	Ponce Paramedical College Mr Leopoldo Vega, Director *Chair's #: (787) 848-1719*	Calle Acacia L-15 Ponce 00731				TCH	PBL			Publication withheld			
027	Ponce Tech School Mrs Roxana Lanause, Director *Chair's #: (787) 844-7940*	Calle Salud #14 Ponce 00731				TCH	PBL	15	12	27	24	46	16
045	PR Tech & Beauty College Mr Angel Arriaga Rivera, Dir *Chair's #: (787) 785-3119*	Box 849 Bayamon 00621				CC	PBL			Publication withheld			

Explanation of footnotes on page x

School Code	Name of School, Director of Program, and Phone Number	Street Address, City or Town and Zip Code	Footnotes	Type of Program	NLNAC Accreditation as of January 31, 1999	Administrative Control	Financial Support (principal source)	Number of Months in Program	Educational Requirements for Entering Adult Program	Enrollments as of October 15, 1998	Admissions Aug. 1, 1997 - July 31, 1998	Graduations Aug. 1, 1997 - July 31, 1998	Fall Admissions Aug. 1, 1998 - Dec. 31, 1998
	PUERTO RICO												
	- Continued												
089	Ramirez Coll of Business and Tech Ms Evelyn Mercado Ruiz, Dir *Chair's #: (787) 763-3120*	Ave Ponce De Leon #70 Hato Rey 00919				TCH	PBL			Publication withheld			
015	Republica de Costa Rica Voc HS Mrs Vilma Gracia, Nsg Teacher *Chair's #: (787) 743-4113*	PO Box 5759 Caguas 00726				TCH	PBL			Publication withheld			
087	Rosslyn Training Academy Ms Rosin Gonzalez, Pres *Chair's #: (787) 868-2902*	213 Calle Paz Aguada 00602				TCH	PVT			Publication withheld			
007	Ryder Memorial Hosp PN Program Mrs Sara Cruz Rivera, Dir *Chair's #: (787) 852-0768 Ext 4588*	PO Box 859 Humacao 00792			A	TCH	PVT	12	12	53	53	42	53
010	Santiago Veve HS-Dr Urgell Voc Prog Ms Hilda Collado Baez, Dir *Chair's #: (787) 863-0424*	Fajardo 00648				SEC	PBL			Publication withheld			
014	Thomas C Ongay Voc HS Mr German Figueroa, Dir *Chair's #: (787) 785-3414*	PO Box 254 Bayamon 00956				SEC	PBL			Publication withheld			
063	Trinity College Ms Elizabeth Perez, Dir *Chair's #: (787) 848--5739 Ext 224*	Avenida Hostos 16 Box 3013 Ponce 00724				TCH	PVT			Publication withheld			
048	Universal Technology Coll of PR Inc Ms Esther Santiago, Director *Chair's #: (787) 882-2065*	Calle Comercio Box 1955 Aguadilla 00605				TCH	PVT			Publication withheld			
	RHODE ISLAND												
	1 Program in 1 School												
001	Community College of Rhode Island Mrs Doris A Fournier, Chair *Chair's #: (401) 333-7217*	Louisquisset Pike Lincoln 02865	7		A	CC	PBL			Data reported w/AD prog			
	SOUTH CAROLINA												
	24 Programs in 24 Schools												
050	Aiken Technical College Mrs Ruth C Croom, Coordinator *Chair's #: (803) 593-9231 Ext 1404*	PO Drawer 696 Aiken 29802				TCH	PBL			Publication withheld			
024	Applied Technology Education Campus Mrs Sharon Clyburn, Coord *Chair's #: (803) 425-8982*	874 Vocational Lane Camden 29020		HSE		TCH TCH	PBL PBL			Publication withheld			
052	Central Carolina Tech Coll Mrs Laurie Harden, Dept Chair *Chair's #: (803) 778-7811*	506 North Guignard Dr Sumter 29150				TCH	PBL	12	12	19	20	11	20

Explanation of footnotes on page x

School Code	Name of School, Director of Program, and Phone Number	Street Address / City or Town and Zip Code	Footnotes	Type of Program	NLNAC Accreditation as of January 31, 1999	Administrative Control	Financial Support (principal source)	Number of Months in Program	Educational Requirements for Entering Adult Program	Enrollments as of October 15, 1998	Admissions Aug. 1, 1997 - July 31, 1998	Graduations Aug. 1, 1997 - July 31, 1998	Fall Admissions Aug. 1, 1998 - Dec. 31, 1998
	SOUTH CAROLINA **- Continued**												
012	Cherokee Technology Center Mrs Janet Carroll, Coord *Chair's #: (864) 489-3191*	Box 3206 Cherokee Ave Gaffney 29340				TCH	PBL			Publication withheld			
033	Chester Sch of PN Mrs Kathy Nance, Coord *Chair's #: (803) 377-1991*	121 Columbia St Chester 29706				TCH	PBL	12	12	12	21	7	22
053	Chesterfield Marlboro Tech Coll Mrs Carolyn Wallace, Coord *Chair's #: (843) 921-6966*	PO Drawer 1007 Cheraw 29520				TCH	PBL			Publication withheld			
017	Conway Sch of PN Mrs Gail H Moss, Coord *Chair's #: (843) 365-5534 Ext 231*	335 Four Mile Rd Conway 29526	HSE		A A	SEC SEC	PBL PBL	18	12	0 29	0 29	0 15	0 33
049	Florence Darlington Tech College Mrs Anne-Marie Goff, Dept Head *Chair's #: (843) 661-8147*	PO Box 100548 Florence 29501	7		A	TCH	PVT	12	12	27	39	9	0
004	Greenville Tech College Mrs Lydia Dunaway, Dept Head *Chair's #: (864) 250 8342*	PO Box 5616 Greenville 29606			A	TCH	PBL	12	12	54	63	43	31
018	Hartsville High Sch Mrs Athena Moree, Coord *Chair's #: (843) 383-3168*	701 Lewellyn Ave Hartsville 29550				SEC	PBL	12	12	14	21	14	19
046	Horry-Georgetown Tech Coll PN Prog Mrs Mary Harper, Dept Head *Chair's #: (843) 546-8406*	4003 S Fraser St Georgetown 29440			A	TCH	PBL			38	35	24	34
005	Lancaster Sch of PN Ms Denise Roberts, Coord *Chair's #: (803) 285-7404 Ext 238*	625 Normandy Rd Lancaster 29720				TCH	PBL	12	12	18	17	12	17
025	Marion Sch of PN Mrs Mary L Pool, Coord *Chair's #: (843) 423-9800*	PO Box 890 Marion 29571	HSE			TCH TCH	PBL PBL	18 18	12 12	44 1	22 3	12 0	28 1
040	Midlands Technical College Dr Margaret Rodes, Dept Head *Chair's #: (803) 822-3320*	PO Box 2408 Columbia 29202	7		A	TCH	PBL	12	12	66	77	45	46
047	Newberry County Career Ctr PN Prog Mrs Elaine Allcut, Coord *Chair's #: (803) 321-2674*	3413 Main St Newberry 29108	HSE			SEC SEC	PBL PBL			Publication withheld			
028	Oconee Sch of PN-F P Hamilton Career Mrs Jane Finfrock, Coord *Chair's #: (864) 885-5011 Ext 28*	100 Vocational Dr Seneca 29672	HSE			TCH TCH	PBL PBL	18 18	12 12	31 4	28 4	11 1	19 4

Explanation of footnotes on page x

School Code	Name of School, Director of Program, and Phone Number	Street Address / City or Town and Zip Code	Footnotes	Type of Program	NLNAC Accreditation as of January 31, 1999	Administrative Control	Financial Support (principal source)	Number of Months in Program	Educational Requirements for Entering Adult Program	Enrollments as of October 15, 1998	Admissions Aug. 1, 1997 - July 31, 1998	Graduations Aug. 1, 1997 - July 31, 1998	Fall Admissions Aug. 1, 1998 - Dec. 31, 1998
	SOUTH CAROLINA												
	- Continued												
044	Orangeburg Calhoun Tech College Mrs Sandra Dewitt, Dept Head *Chair's #: (803) 535-1343*	3250 St Mathews Rd NE Orangeburg 29115			A	TCH	PBL	12	12	40	35	22	34
030	Piedmont Tech College Mrs Lena Warren, Dean *Chair's #: (864) 941-8536*	Emerald Rd, Drawer 1467 Greenwood 29646				TCH	PBL			Publication withheld			
001	Roper Hosp Mrs Beth Stone, Coord *Chair's #: (843) 763-2699*	316 Calhoun St Charleston 29401				HSP	PVT			Publication withheld			
013	Spartanburg Tech College Ms Linda Hayes, Dept Head *Chair's #: (864) 591-3855*	Drawer 4386 Spartanburg 29305				TCH	PBL			Publication withheld			
045	Tech College of the Lowcountry Dr Patricia Slachta, Dept Head *Chair's #: (843) 525-8267*	PO Box 1288 Beaufort 29902	7		A	TCH	PBL	12	12	27	30	18	27
014	Tri County Tech College Mrs Lynn M Lollis, Dept Head *Chair's #: (864) 646-8361 Ext 2468*	PO Box 587 Pendleton 29670				TCH	PBL	12	12	25	23	20	19
051	Trident Tech College Ms Muriel Horton, Dean *Chair's #: (843) 574-6138*	Box 118067 Charleston 29423			A	TCH	PBL	12	12	49	60	42	48
	SOUTH DAKOTA												
	2 Programs in 2 Schools												
004	Lake Area Tech Inst Mrs Julie Hanson, Dept Head *Chair's #: (605) 882-5284 Ext 286*	230 11th St NE Watertown 57201			A	TCH	PBL	11	12	34	34	27	34
006	Western Dakota Voc-Tech Inst Ms Donna Belitz, Coord *Chair's #: (605) 394-4034 Ext 112*	800 Michelson Dr Rapid City 57701				TCH	PBL	11	12	26	32	23	40
	TENNESSEE												
	25 Programs in 25 Schools												
021	Appalachian Reg PN Prog Mr Annabelle Harvey, Coord *Chair's #: (423) 525-3219*	PO Box 419 Jackboro 37757				TCH	PBL	0	12	81	99	67	55
044	Baptist Memorial Coll Hlth Sciences Ms Valarie Vendetta Tatum, Chair *Chair's #: (901) 227-4409*	1003 Monroe Ave Memphis 38104	1			COL	PVT	11	12	49	51	7	35
702	Blount Memorial Hosp Ms Polly Evans, Director *Chair's #: (423) 982 3134*	907 E Lamar Alexander Pky Maryville 37801				SEC	PVT	11	12	22	24	21	0

Explanation of footnotes on page x

School Code	Name of School, Director of Program, and Phone Number	Street Address, City or Town and Zip Code	Footnotes	Type of Program	NLNAC Accreditation as of January 31, 1999	Administrative Control	Financial Support (principal source)	Number of Months in Program	Educational Requirements for Entering Adult Program	Enrollments as of October 15, 1998	Admissions Aug. 1, 1997 - July 31, 1998	Graduations Aug. 1, 1997 - July 31, 1998	Fall Admissions Aug. 1, 1998 - Dec. 31, 1998
	TENNESSEE												
	- Continued												
646	Bristol TN PN Prog Mrs Barbara DeBusk, Director *Chair's #: (423) 652-9206*	325 Mcdowell St SlaterCenter Bristol City 37620				SEC	PBL	11	12	21	39	16	0
037	Chattanooga State Tech Comm College Mrs Donna Roddy, Dir *Chair's #: (423) 697-4447 Ext 4491*	4501 Amnicola Hwy Chattanooga 37406				CC	PBL	12	12	39	68	47	37
640	Four Rivers Regional PN Prog Mrs Belinda Douglas, Coord *Chair's #: (901) 475-2526 Ext 18*	PO Box 249 Covington 38019				TCH	PBL			Publication withheld			
022	Jackson Regional PN Program Ms Barbara Avent, Coord *Chair's #: (901) 424-0691 Ext 120*	2468 Westover Rd Jackson 38301				TCH	PBL	12	12	96	127	77	69
002	Methodist Hospitals of Memphis Mrs Janie Daniells,Dir *Chair's #: (901) 726-8861*	251 South Claybrook Memphis 38104				HSP	PVT	12	12	46	54	16	0
015	Nashville Memorial Hosp Mrs Anna House, Director *Chair's #: (615) 865-3440*	612 W Due West Ave Madison 37115				HSP	PVT	12	12	22	24	16	24
011	South Central Reg PN Ms Vicki Barnette, Dir *Chair's #: (615) 424-4014*	PO Box 614 1244 E College Pulaski 38778				TCH	PBL			Publication withheld			
005	Sumner County PN Prog Mrs Cathy Eden Ammerman, Supv *Chair's #: (615) 452-4210 Ext 5164*	PO Box 1558 Gallatin 37066				SEC	PBL	11	12	21	24	17	22
038	TN Tech Center Mrs Anita Hemmeter, Dir *Chair's #: (423) 546-5567 Ext 136*	1100 Liberty St Knoxville 37919				TCH	PBL	12	12	64	71	34	35
034	TN Tech Center Mrs Sandra Wakefield, Dir *Chair's #: (615) 741-1241 Ext 34*	100 White Bridge Rd Nashville 37209				TCH	PBL			Publication withheld			
033	TN Tech Center Ms Roberta McCord, Director *Chair's #: (931) 473-5587 Ext 246*	241 Voc Tech Dr McMinnville 37110				TCH	PBL			Publication withheld			
031	TN Tech Center Mrs Terri Barnett Blevins, Dir *Chair's #: (423) 547-2590 Ext 412*	1500 Arney St PO Box 789 Elizabethton 37644				TCH	PBL	12	12	108	73	38	110
030	TN Tech Center Mrs Laura Travis, Coord *Chair's #: (615) 441-6220 Ext 110*	740 Hwy 46 Dickson 37055				TCH	PBL	12	12	43	63	46	0

Explanation of footnotes on page x

School Code	Name of School, Director of Program, and Phone Number	Street Address City or Town and Zip Code	Footnotes	Type of Program	NLNAC Accreditation as of January 31, 1999	Administrative Control	Financial Support (principal source)	Number of Months in Program	Educational Requirements for Entering Adult Program	Enrollments as of October 15, 1998	Admissions Aug. 1, 1997 - July 31, 1998	Graduations Aug. 1, 1997 - July 31, 1998	Fall Admissions Aug. 1, 1998 - Dec. 31, 1998
	TENNESSEE												
	- Continued												
029	TN Tech Center Ms Linda Bilbrey, Dir *Chair's #: (931) 484-7502 Ext 38*	PO Box 2959 910 N Miller Ave Crossville 38557				TCH	PBL	12	12	37	48	26	24
028	TN Tech Center Mrs Linda Nein, Coord *Chair's #: (423)744-2814 Ext 0215*	PO Box 848 Athens 37303				TCH	PBL	12	12	42	45	30	32
026	TN Tech Center Ms Linda Wier, Coord *Chair's #: (931) 685-5013 Ext 119*	1405 Madison Ave Shelbyville 37160				TCH	PBL	12	12	44	44	32	39
024	TN Tech Center Ms Karen McGill, Coord *Chair's #: (423) 586-5771 Ext 264*	821 W Louise St Box 130 Morristown 37813				TCH	PBL	12	12	75	86	64	46
023	TN Tech Center Mrs Patrice Gilliam, Coord *Chair's #: (931) 403-3116*	PO Box 219 Livingston 38570				TCH	PBL	12	12	76	85	72	50
004	TN Tech Center Mr Theresa Isom, Coord *Chair's #: (901) 543-6126*	550 Alabama Ave Memphis 38105				TCH	PBL			Publication withheld			
025	TN Technology Center Ms Alice B McCutcheon, Coord *Chair's #: (901) 644-7365 Ext 129*	312 S Wilson St Paris 38242				TCH	PBL	12	12	45	56	16	29
008	Weakley Co Voc Center Mrs Gwendolyn Scarborough, Dir *Chair's #: (901) 364-5481*	8250 Hwy 22 Dresden 38225				TCH	PBL	12	12	24	24	20	12
	TEXAS												
	121 Programs in 74 Schools												
034	Alvin Comm College Ms Judy Siefert, Chair *Chair's #: (281) 388-4691*	3110 Mustang Rd Alvin 77511				CC	PBL	12	12	22	28	19	4
001	Amarillo College Ms Delores Thompson. Coordinator *Chair's #: (806) 354-6018*	Box 447 Amarillo 79178				CC	PBL	12	12	72	77	28	32
052	AMEDD Center School Dr Lynn Connelly, Chief Dept of Nsg *Chair's #: (210) 221-8336 Ext 8715*	2250 Stanley Rd MCCS-HNP Ft Sam Houston 78234	5			GOV	PBL			625	681	526	325
065	Angelina College Ms Kathy Bredberg, Dir *Chair's #: (409) 384-1994*	1275 Marvin Hancock Dr Jasper 75951				CC	PBL	12	12	16	16	0	16

Explanation of footnotes on page x

TEXAS

- Continued

School Code	Name of School, Director of Program, and Phone Number	Street Address / City or Town and Zip Code	Footnotes	Type of Program	NLNAC Accreditation as of January 31, 1999	Administrative Control	Financial Support (principal source)	Number of Months in Program	Educational Requirements for Entering Adult Program	Enrollments as of October 15, 1998	Admissions Aug. 1, 1997 - July 31, 1998	Graduations Aug. 1, 1997 - July 31, 1998	Fall Admissions Aug. 1, 1998 - Dec. 31, 1998
024	Angelina College Div of Hlth Careers Ms Kathleen Hall, Inteim Dir *Chair's #: (409) 633-5265 Ext 241*	PO Box 1768 Lufkin 75901	7			CC	PBL			Data reported w/AD prog			
061	Austin Comm Coll Ms Yvonne VanDyke, Coord *Chair's #: (512) 223-6116*	PO Box 835 Fredericksburg 78624				CC	PBL			Publication withheld			
691	Austin Comm College Mrs Yvonne Vandyke, Dept Coord *Chair's #: (512) 223-6116*	1020 Grove Austin 78741			A	CC	PBL	15	12	90	39	29	56
094	Baptist Hlth System Mrs Maxine Cadena, Director *Chair's #: (210) 297-1250*	111 Dallas San Antonio 78205				HSP	PVT			Publication withheld			
030	Baptist Hlth System (Evening) Mrs Maxine Cadena, Director *Chair's #: (210)297-9100*	111 Dallas St San Antonio 78205				HSP	PVT			Publication withheld			
028	Bee Co College-Alice Extension Mrs Iva Burgan, Dir *Chair's #: (512) 664-1492*	704 Coyote Trail Alice 78332				CC	PBL			Publication withheld			
064	Bee Co College-Kingsville Branch Ms Noemi Arsona Peterson, Dir *Chair's #: (512) 593-2636*	PO Box 2140 Station I Kingsville 78363				CC	PBL			Publication withheld			
659	Bee County College Mrs Betty Sims, Dir *Chair's #: (512) 358-3130 Ext 2280*	3800 Charco Rd Beeville 78102				CC	PBL			33	35	24	0
756	Blinn College Ms Mary Arnold, Dir *Chair's #: (409) 821-0202*	902 College Ave Brenham 77833				CC	PBL			Publication withheld			
762	Blinn College at Bryan Mrs Mary Arnold, Director *Chair's #: (409) 821-0203 Ext 38*	PO Box 6030 Bryan 77805	7			CC	PBL			Data reported w/AD prog			
604	Brazosport Comm College VN Prog Mrs Pamela Gwin, Dir *Chair's #: (409) 230-3290*	500 College Dr Lake Jackson 77566				CC	PBL	11	12	24	27	12	28
664	Central Texas College Dr Shirley Robertson, Chair *Chair's #: (254) 526-1300*	6200 W Central TX Expresswa Killeen 76542				TCH	PBL	12	12	75	84	82	12
783	Central Texas College-Brady Ext Dr Elaine E Hayes, Chair *Chair's #: (915) 597-2901 Ext 466*	Nine Rd Box 1361 Brady 76825				CC	PBL			Data with #664			

School Code	Name of School, Director of Program, and Phone Number	Street Address / City or Town and Zip Code		Footnotes	Type of Program	NLNAC Accreditation as of January 31, 1999	Administrative Control	Financial Support (principal source)	Number of Months in Program	Educational Requirements for Entering Adult Program	Enrollments as of October 15, 1998	Admissions Aug. 1, 1997 - July 31, 1998	Graduations Aug. 1, 1997 - July 31, 1998	Fall Admissions Aug. 1, 1998 - Dec. 31, 1998
	TEXAS													
	- Continued													
081	Childress Reg Med Center Ms Kathy Lindley, Dir *Chair's #: (940) 937-7021*	PO Box 1030 Childress	79202				HSP	PBL			Publication withheld			
613	Cisco Jr College-Abilene Mrs Jackolyn Morgan, Dir *Chair's #: (915) 673-4567 Ext 236*	841 N Judge Ely Blvd Abilene	79601			A	CC	PBL	12	12	65	68	53	23
649	Clarendon College VN Program Ms Vickie Moore, Dir *Chair's #: (806) 874-3571 Ext 44*	Box 968 Clarendon	79226				TCH	PBL			37	35	35	0
003	Del Mar College Mrs Bertha Almendarez, Chair *Chair's #: (512) 886-1394*	Baldwin & Ayers Corpus Christi	78404				CC	PBL			79	70	56	39
713	Delta Career Inst Voc Prog Mrs Charlotte Vannett, Director *Chair's #: (409) 833-6161 Ext 411*	1310 Pennsylvania Beaumont	77001				TCH	PVT	12	12	34	49	36	17
911	E & K Voc Nursing Prog Miss Paulette Potter, Dir *Chair's #: (972) 630-6783*	5415 Maple Ave Suite 114 Dallas	75235				TCH	PVT			Publication withheld			
652	El Centro College Ms Frances Warrick, Coord *Chair's #: (214) 860-2288*	Main & Lamar Dallas	75202			A	CC	PBL			30	42	32	29
066	El Paso Comm Coll Dr Paula Michell, Div Dean *Chair's #: (915) 831-4030*	PO Box 20500 El Paso	79778				CC	PBL			Publication withheld			
006	El Paso Comm College Dr Paula Mitchell, Dean *Chair's #: (915) 831-4030*	PO Box 20500 El Paso	79998		7		CC	PBL			Data reported with/AD pro			
005	Extended Hlth Education Ms Gloria Edwards, Dir *Chair's #: (817) 261-1594*	1619 West Division Suite O Arlington	76012				IND	PBL	12	12	52	48	19	28
070	Fort Duncan Medical Center Mrs Fe Sandoval, Dir *Chair's #: (830) 773-5321 Ext 576*	350 S Adams St Eagle Pass	78852				HSP	PBL			Publication withheld			
606	Frank Philips College-VN Prog Mrs Marilyn Wood, Dir *Chair's #: (806) 274-5311 Ext 745*	Box 5118 Borger	79008				TCH	PBL			Publication withheld			
665	Galveston Comm College Mrs Elizabeth Michel, Asst Dean *Chair's #: (409) 763-6551 Ext 387*	4015 Ave Q Galveston	77550				CC	PBL	12	12	19	22	23	22

Explanation of footnotes on page x

School Code	Name of School, Director of Program, and Phone Number	Street Address / City or Town and Zip Code		Footnotes	Type of Program	NLNAC Accreditation as of January 31, 1999	Administrative Control	Financial Support (principal source)	Number of Months in Program	Educational Requirements for Entering Adult Program	Enrollments as of October 15, 1998	Admissions Aug. 1, 1997 - July 31, 1998	Graduations Aug. 1, 1997 - July 31, 1998	Fall Admissions Aug. 1, 1998 - Dec. 31, 1998
	TEXAS													
	- Continued													
639	Grayson County College Mrs Jenann Allen, Dir *Chair's #: (903) 786-4468 Ext 17*	6101 Grayson Dr Denison	75021				CC	PBL	12	12	43	38	34	0
917	Health Care Training Center Mrs Maria Flecher, President *Chair's #: (210) 687-8138*	2715 Cornerstone Blvd Edinburg	78539				IND	PVT			10	12	10	0
089	Hill College Ms Sharon Allen, Dir *Chair's #: (254) 582-2555 Ext 281*	PO Box 619 Hillsboro	76645				CC	PBL	12	12	17	24	23	0
631	Hill College-Cleburne Ext Ms Paula Eubanks, Dir *Chair's #: (817) 645-7522*	1505 W Henderson Cleburne	76031				TCH	PBL			48	48	48	24
077	Hill College-Clifton Ms Helen M Amundson, Director *Chair's #: (254) 675-6700*	101 S Ave "T" Clifton	76634				CC	PBL	12	12	12	12	10	12
021	Houston Comm College Ms Dorothy Collins, Chair *Chair's #: (713) 718-7332*	3100 Shenandoah Houston	77021				CC	PBL			Publication withheld			
738	Howard College Mrs June Stone, Director *Chair's #: (915) 264-5067*	1001 Birdwell Ln Big Spring	79720				CC	PBL	12	12	17	17	15	17
012	Howard College-San Angelo Mrs Donna Rutledge, Dir *Chair's #: (915) 947-9516 Ext 23*	3197 Executive Dr San Angelo	76904		HSE		CC CC	PBL PBL	12 24	12 12	43 0	38 1	29 0	43 0
063	Inst for Hlth Career Development Ms Loretta Mahaffey, Director *Chair's #: (817) 534-0200 Ext 116*	2400 Circle Drive Suite 100 Ft Worth	76119				HSP	PBL			Publication withheld			
653	Joe G Davis Sch of VN Mrs Barbara Bohanon, Director *Chair's #: (409) 291-4544*	3000 1-45 Huntsville	77340				HSP	PBL	12	12	10	15	17	15
638	John Peter Smith Sch Ms Loretta Mahaffey, Dir *Chair's #: (817) 534-0200 Ext 116*	1500 S Main St Fort Worth	76104				HSP	PBL			Publication withheld			
774	Kilgore College-Longview Ms Barbara Brush, Dir *Chair's #: (903) 753-2642 Ext 24*	300 S High St Longview	75601				CC	PBL			57	66	47	32
029	Kingwood College Mrs Thelma Bowie, Dir *Chair's #: (281) 312-1647*	20000 Kingwood Dr Kingwood	77339				CC	PBL	12	12	56	68	56	33

Explanation of footnotes on page x

School Code	Name of School, Director of Program, and Phone Number	Street Address, City or Town and Zip Code		Footnotes	Type of Program	NLNAC Accreditation as of January 31, 1999	Administrative Control	Financial Support (principal source)	Number of Months in Program	Educational Requirements for Entering Adult Program	Enrollments as of October 15, 1998	Admissions Aug. 1, 1997 - July 31, 1998	Graduations Aug. 1, 1997 - July 31, 1998	Fall Admissions Aug. 1, 1998 - Dec. 31, 1998
	TEXAS													
	- Continued													
772	Lamar Univ at Orange Sch of Voc Nsg Mrs Gina Simar, Dir *Chair's #: (409) 882-3311*	410 Front St Orange	77630				CC	PBL			84	96	72	48
010	Lamar Univ-Port Arthur Ext Ms Mary Mulliner, Coord *Chair's #: (409) 984-6362*	PO Box 310 Pt Arthur	77640				CC	PBL			Publication withheld			
614	Laredo Comm Coll Ms Carolyn Otero, Chair *Chair's #: (956) 721-5255*	W End Washington St Laredo	78040				CC	PBL			33	36	33	0
755	Lee College Voc Nsg Prog Dr Lorena Maher, Chair *Chair's #: (281) 425-6449*	PO Box 818 Baytown	77522				CC	PBL	12	12	35	40	35	35
097	McLennan Comm College (Career Ladd Mrs Alice Myers, Dir *Chair's #: (254) 299-8349*	1400 College Dr Waco	76708	7			CC	PBL			Data reported w/AD prog			
699	McLennan Comm College (Trad Prog) Mrs Leila Clark, Dir *Chair's #: (254) 299-8370*	1400 College Dr Waco	76708				CC	PBL			Publication withheld			
035	Memorial Hosp-Memorial City Sch of V Mrs Judith M Farmer, Director *Chair's #: (713) 932-3799*	920 Frostwood Houston	77024				HSP	PVT	12	12	36	44	40	0
692	Midland College Mrs Susan Jones, Dir *Chair's #: (915) 685-4600*	3600 N Garfield Midland	79701				CC	PBL			Publication withheld			
696	Midland College-Fort Stockton Ext Mrs Helen Dionne, Director *Chair's #: (915) 336-6541*	400 South Young Fort Stockton	79735				CC	PBL	12	12	15	15	9	15
915	Montgomery College Mrs Thelma Bowie, Dir *Chair's #: (409) 273-7030*	2000 Kingwood Dr Kingwood	77339				CC	PBL	12	12	24	24	23	24
650	Navarro College Dr Judy Howden, Dir *Chair's #: (903) 874-6501 Ext 255*	Box 1170 Corsicana	75110				CC	PBL			Publication withheld			
082	Navarro College-Mexia Ext Dr Judy Howden, Director *Chair's #: (903) 874-6501*	PO Box 1132 Mexia	76667				CC	PBL			Publication withheld			
050	Navarro College-Waxahachie Ext Dr Judy Howden, Dir *Chair's #: (903) 874-6501 Ext 213*	1900 John Arden Dr Waxahachie	75165				CC	PBL			Publication withheld			

Explanation of footnotes on page x

School Code	Name of School, Director of Program, and Phone Number	Street Address / City or Town and Zip Code		Footnotes	Type of Program	NLNAC Accreditation as of January 31, 1999	Administrative Control	Financial Support (principal source)	Number of Months in Program	Educational Requirements for Entering Adult Program	Enrollments as of October 15, 1998	Admissions Aug. 1, 1997 - July 31, 1998	Graduations Aug. 1, 1997 - July 31, 1998	Fall Admissions Aug. 1, 1998 - Dec. 31, 1998
	TEXAS													
	- Continued													
786	North Central TX College Ms Carol Brown, Coord Chair's #: (940) 668-4291 Ext 322	1525 W California Gainesville	76240				CC	PBL	12	12	81	106	78	90
041	North Harris College Mrs Margaret Aalund, Director Chair's #: (281) 618-5751	2700 W W Thorne Dr Houston	77073	7			CC	PBL			Data reported w/AD prog			
720	Northeast TX Comm College Mrs Cynthia Amerson, Director Chair's #: (903) 572-1911 Ext 356	PO Box 1307 Mt Pleasant	75455				CC	PBL			36	36	24	37
046	Odessa College Dr Carol Boswell, Chair Chair's #: (915) 335-6463	201 W University Odessa	79760	7			CC	PBL			Data reported w /AD prog			
711	Odessa College-Andrews Ext Ms Patricia Bayless, Dept Chair Chair's #: (915) 524-4022	405 N W 3rd Andrews	79714				CC	PBL	12		25	30	26	30
725	Odessa College-Kermit Ext Mrs Anne Mitchell, Director Chair's #: (915)	821 Jeffee Dr Kermit	79745				TCH	PBL			Publication withheld			
909	Panola College Mrs Varonica Dickerson, Chair Chair's #: (830) 694-4007	PO Box 647 Jefferson	75657	7			CC	PBL			Data with w/AD prog			
769	Panola College Mrs Varonica Dickerson, Chair Chair's #: (903) 694-4007	820 West Panola Carthage	75633	7			CC	PBL			Data reportedw/AD prog			
059	Panola College Mrs Varonica Dickerson, Chair Chair's #: (409) 598-2730	PO Box 1863 Center	75935	7			CC	PBL			Data reported w\AD prog			
718	Paris Jr College (Ladder Prog) Mrs Virginia Holmes, Director Chair's #: (903) 782-0734	2400 Clarksville St Paris	75460				CC	PBL			Data reported w/AD prog			
905	Ranger College-Graham Ext Mrs Elaine Gates, Dir Chair's #: (940) 549-4678	Box 837 Graham	76046				CC	PBL			15	15	13	15
037	Ranger Jr College-Brownwood Ext Ms Kathy Brown, Dir Chair's #: (915) 643-3852	PO Box 837 Brownwood	76801				CC	PBL			Publication withheld			
038	San Jacinto College-North, Sch of VN Mrs Beverly Smith, Dir Chair's #: (281) 459-7114	5800 Uvalde Houston	77049				CC	PBL	12	12	92	72	36	58

Explanation of footnotes on page x

TEXAS
- Continued

School Code	Name of School, Director of Program, and Phone Number	Street Address, City or Town and Zip Code	Footnotes	Type of Program	NLNAC Accreditation as of January 31, 1999	Administrative Control	Financial Support (principal source)	Number of Months in Program	Educational Requirements for Entering Adult Program	Enrollments as of October 15, 1998	Admissions Aug. 1, 1997 - July 31, 1998	Graduations Aug. 1, 1997 - July 31, 1998	Fall Admissions Aug. 1, 1998 - Dec. 31, 1998
712	San Jacinto College-South Campus Mrs Joyce Pfleeger, Chair Chair's #: (281) 922-3405	13735 Beamer Rd Houston 77089				CC	PBL	12	12	95	119	71	61
708	Schreiner College VN Prog Mrs Rosemary Pullin, Director Chair's #: (830) 792-7385	Box 4491 Kerrville 78028				COL	PVT	12	12	54	60	50	30
741	South Plains College Mrs Sue Ann Lopez, Dir Chair's #: (806) 894-9611 Ext 2390	1401 College Ave Levelland 79336				CC	PBL			Publication withheld			
704	South Plains College-Lubbock Ext Ms Korbi Berryhill, Coord Chair's #: (806) 747-0576 Ext 4622	1302 Main Lubbock 79401				TCH	PBL			45	90	46	45
048	South Plains College-Plainview Ext Mrs Donna Womble, Director Chair's #: (806) 291-4391	708 Yonkers Plainview 79072				CC	PBL			Publication withheld			
083	South Texas Comm Coll Ms Celinda De Luna, Chair Chair's #: (956) 969-5467	1401 East 8th St Weslasco 78596				CC	PVT			Publication withheld			
916	South Texas Comm College Ms Melva Trevino, Chair Chair's #: (956) 618-8341	3201 W Pecan Blvd McAllen 78502				CC	PVT			Publication withheld			
914	Southwest Texas Jr College Mrs Suzanne Rue, Director Chair's #: (830) 591-7316	207 Wildcat Dr. Del Rio 78842				CC	PBL	9	12	18	18	15	18
728	Southwest Texas Jr College Mrs Suzanne Rue, Director Chair's #: (830) 591-7316	Box 70 Garner Field Rd Uvalde 78801				CC	PBL	9	12	27	35	29	28
022	St Philips College Mrs Annie Brown, Dir Chair's #: (210) 531-3415 Ext 3427	1801 Martin Luther King San Antonio 78203			A	CC	PBL	12	12	80	161	108	85
658	St Philips College-New Braunfels Ext Mrs Susan Bell, Coord Chair's #: (830) 606-9111 Ext 244	610 N Houston St New Braunfels 78130				CC	PBL			Publication withheld			
743	Sul Ross Univ Ms Glenda Klassen, Dir Chair's #: (915) 837-8171	Box C-58 Alpine 79832				COL	PBL			Publication withheld			
700	Temple Jr College VN Prog Mrs Virginia Leak, Director Chair's #: (254) 298-8666	2600 S First Street Temple 76504				CC	PBL	12	12	59	72	33	0

Explanation of footnotes on page x

TEXAS
- Continued

School Code	Name of School, Director of Program, and Phone Number	Street Address / City or Town and Zip Code	Footnotes	Type of Program	NLNAC Accreditation as of January 31, 1999	Administrative Control	Financial Support (principal source)	Number of Months in Program	Educational Requirements for Entering Adult Program	Enrollments as of October 15, 1998	Admissions Aug. 1, 1997 - July 31, 1998	Graduations Aug. 1, 1997 - July 31, 1998	Fall Admissions Aug. 1, 1998 - Dec. 31, 1998
092	Texarkana Comm College Mrs Carol Hodgson, Chair Chair's #: (903) 838-4541 Ext 401	2500 N Robinson Rd Box 9150 Texarkana 75501				CC	PBL	12	12	85	94	87	55
045	Texas Career Inc Ms Kiska Varela, Dir Chair's #: (210) 308-8584 Ext 33	1015 Jackson Keller San Antonio 78213				TCH	PBL			24	20	15	24
020	Texas State Tech Coll-Breckenridge Mrs Jackie Ververs, Coord Chair's #: (915) 235-7388	307 N Breckenridge Breckenridge 76424				TCH	PBL			Publication withheld			
075	Texas State Tech College Mrs Carrie Sanderson, Chair Chair's #: (915) 235-7388 Ext 388	Box 18 Rt3 Sweetwater 79556				TCH	PBL			Publication withheld			
910	The Health Inst of San Antonio Dr Peggy Richardson, Dir Chair's #: (210) 733-3056	6800 Park Ten Blvd Suite 160 San Antonio 78213				TCH	PVT			121	148	118	70
031	Tomball College Mrs Kathleen Emmite, Dir Chair's #: (281) 357-3720	30555 Tomball Parkway Tomball 77375	7			CC	PBL			Data reported w/AD prog			
908	Tri City Comm Hosp Sch of Voc Nsg Mrs Donna Zimmerman, Dir Chair's #: (830) 769-3515 Ext 1065	Hwy 97 E PO Box 189 Jourdanton 78026				HSP	PVT	12	12	11	12	11	0
901	Trinity Valley Comm Coll Mrs Helen Reid, Dean Chair's #: (972) 932-4309	PO Box 2530 Palestine 75802				CC	PBL	0	12	36	35	33	36
095	Trinity Valley Comm College Mrs Helen Reid, Dean Chair's #: (972) 932-4309	800 Hwy 243 W Kaufman 75142				CC	PBL	12	12	19	24	21	0
752	Tyler County Hosp Mrs Eva Stanley, Director Chair's #: (409) 283-8141 Ext 246	1100 W Bluff Woodville 75979				HSP	PBL	12	12	14	15	15	0
004	Tyler Jr College Ms Jean Boyer, Coord Chair's #: (903) 586-3000	501 S S Ragsdale Jacksonville 75766				CC	PVT			Publication withheld			
017	Tyler Jr College VN Prog Mrs Adelia Miller, Director Chair's #: (903) 510-2471	Box 9020 Tyler 75711				CC	PBL	12	10	59	60	50	60
084	Univ of Texas-Brownsville Ms Gloria Spencer, Dir Chair's #: (956) 544-3865 Ext 1874	80 Ft Brown Brownsville 78520				COL	PBL			Publication withheld			

Explanation of footnotes on page x

School Code	Name of School, Director of Program, and Phone Number	Street Address / City or Town and Zip Code	Footnotes	Type of Program	NLNAC Accreditation as of January 31, 1999	Administrative Control	Financial Support (principal source)	Number of Months in Program	Educational Requirements for Entering Adult Program	Enrollments as of October 15, 1998	Admissions Aug. 1, 1997 - July 31, 1998	Graduations Aug. 1, 1997 - July 31, 1998	Fall Admissions Aug. 1, 1998 - Dec. 31, 1998
	TEXAS												
	- Continued												
715	Valley Baptist Medical Ctr Mrs Barbara DisBennett, Director *Chair's #: (956) 389-1721*	PO Drawer 2588 Harlingen 78550				HSP	PVT	13	10	27	43	25	39
912	Valley Grande Coll of Hlth and Tech Mrs Ramona Midamba, Director *Chair's #: (956) 973-1945 18*	800 W Railroad, Blgd W Box 8 Westasco 78596				IND	PVT			Publication withheld			
051	Vanguard Inst of Technoloy Ms Alma Carson, Director *Chair's #: (956) 380-3264*	221 N 8th St Edinburg 78539				TCH	PBL			Publication withheld			
018	Vernon Reg Jr College Ms Cathy J Bolton, Director *Chair's #: (940 552-6291 Ext 270*	4400 College Dr Vernon 76384				CC	PBL			Publication withheld			
043	Vernon Reg Jr Wichita Falls Ms Lynn Kalski, Dir *Chair's #: (940) 696-8752 Ext 3222*	4105 Maplewood Ave Wichita Falls 76308				CC	PBL			Publication withheld			
757	Victoria College Ms Marilyn Powell, Dir *Chair's #: (512) 572-6446*	2200 East Red River St Victoria 77901				CC	PBL	12	12	192	203	157	192
015	Victoria College- Gonzales Mrs Faith Darilek, Director *Chair's #: (210) 672-7411*	1103 N Sarah Dewitt Dr Gonzales 78629				CC	PBL			Data with #757			
693	Victoria College-Cuero Ext Ms Deanna L Stenger, Director *Chair's #: (512) 275-6191 Ext 105*	2550 N Esplanade Cuero 77954				CC	PBL			Data with #757			
098	Victoria College-Port Lavaca Ext Mrs Madeline V Garcia, Director *Chair's #: (512) 552-8988*	810 N Ann St Port Lavaca 77979				CC	PBL			Data with #757			
902	Victoria College-Seguin Ext Mrs Gina Burns, Director *Chair's #: (210) 379-2411 Ext 397*	1331 East Court St Seguin 78155				CC	PBL			Data with #757			
074	Victoria College-Yoakum Comm Hosp Mrs Marilyn Powell, Director *Chair's #: (512) 573-3291 Ext 436*	303 Hubbard St, Box 753 Yoakum 77995				CC	PBL			Data with #757			
026	Victoria College-Zelda Allen Mrs Marianne Muehr, Director *Chair's #: (512) 798-2289*	1410 N Texana St Hallettsville 77964				CC	PBL			Data with #757			
025	Weatherford College VN Prog Miss Nita Parsons, Director *Chair's #: (817) 598-6236*	308 E Park PO Box 5033 Weatherford 76086				CC	PBL	12	12	58	67	62	66

School Code	Name of School, Director of Program, and Phone Number	Street Address / City or Town and Zip Code	Footnotes	Type of Program	NLNAC Accreditation as of January 31, 1999	Administrative Control	Financial Support (principal source)	Number of Months in Program	Educational Requirements for Entering Adult Program	Enrollments as of October 15, 1998	Admissions Aug. 1, 1997 - July 31, 1998	Graduations Aug. 1, 1997 - July 31, 1998	Fall Admissions Aug. 1, 1998 - Dec. 31, 1998
TEXAS													
	- Continued												
609	Western Texas College-VN Prog Mrs Diane Beard, Director Chair's #: (915) 573-8511 Ext 227	College Ave Snyder 79549				CC	PBL			Publication withheld			
637	Wharton Co Jr Coll-Richmond Mrs Linda Herrera, Director Chair's #: (281) 232-3775	1601 Main Suite B-03 Richmond 77469				CC	PBL			33	36	18	36
019	Wharton Co Jr College Ms Nelta Maffett, Dir Chair's #: (409) 532-6399	911 Boling Highway Wharton 77488				CC	PBL			Publication withheld			
	UTAH												
	8 Programs in 7 Schools												
007	Coll of Eastern Utah at Price Ms Diana Baker, Dir Chair's #: (435) 613-5261	451 E 400, N Price 84501				CC	PBL	12	12	31	49	44	31
008	Davis Applied Technical Ms Wendy Boren, Coord Chair's #: (801) 593-2331	550 E 300 S Kaysville 84037				TCH	PBL			Publication withheld			
004	Dixie College Mr Kevin Tipton, Dir Chair's #: (435) 652-7730	225 S 700 E St George 84770				CC	PBL	9	12	23	50	20	24
002	Salt Lake Community College Ms Marilyn Little, Coord Chair's #: (801) 957-5704	4600 S Redwood Rd Box 3080 Salt Lake City 84130	7		A	CC	PBL			Data reported w/AD prog			
010	Snow College South Susan Ferguson, Director Chair's #: (435) 896-9728	800 W 200 South Richfield 84701				TCH	PBL	8	12	20	20	20	20
009	Uintah Basin Area Tech Ctr Mr Brett Robbins, Director Chair's #: (801) 722-4523 Ext 114	1100 E Lagoon St PO 124-5 Roosevelt 84066				TCH	PBL			Publication withheld			
001	Utah Valley State College Mrs Karin L Swendsen, Director Chair's #: (801) 222-8190	800 West 1200 South Orem 84058				COL	PBL	8	12	105	106	101	57
005	Weber State University Ms Pamela Rice, Coord Chair's #: (801) 626-6737	3750 Harrison Blvd Ogden 84408			A	COL	PBL			Publication withheld			
	VERMONT												
	4 Programs in 1 School												
003	Vermont Tech College Ms Patricia Menchini, Dir Chair's #: (802) 447-2540	29 Ethan Allen Ave Colchester 05446			A	TCH	PBL			Data with #006			

Explanation of footnotes on page x

School Code	Name of School, Director of Program, and Phone Number	Street Address City or Town and Zip Code		Footnotes	Type of Program	NLNAC Accreditation as of January 31, 1999	Administrative Control	Financial Support (principal source)	Number of Months in Program	Educational Requirements for Entering Adult Program	Enrollments as of October 15, 1998	Admissions Aug. 1, 1997 - July 31, 1998	Graduations Aug. 1, 1997 - July 31, 1998	Fall Admissions Aug. 1, 1998 - Dec. 31, 1998
	VERMONT													
	- Continued													
001	Vermont Tech College Ms Patricia Menchini, Dir *Chair's #: (802) 447-5419*	Bennington	05201			A	TCH	PBL			Data with #006			
006	Vermont Technical College Ms Patricia Menchini, Dir *Chair's #: (802) 447-5419*	PO Box 500 Randolph Center	05061			A	TCH	PBL	10	12	71	101	85	81
002	Vermont Technical College Ms Patricia Menchini, Dir *Chair's #: (802) 254-5570*	30 Maple St Brattleboro	05301			A	TCH	PBL			Data with #006			
	VIRGIN ISLANDS													
	1 Program in 1 School													
900	St Croix Voc Skills Center Mrs Cynthia Vanwingerden, Coord *Chair's #: (340) 778-2216 Ext 234*	21-22-23-Hospital St C'sted St Croix	00820				TCH	PBL	12	12	12	11	8	13
	VIRGINIA													
	58 Programs in 55 Schools													
055	Alexandria City Schs / Alex Hosp Ms Sandra Ballif, Director *Chair's #: (703) 824-6858*	3330 King St Alexandria	22302		HSE		SEC SEC	PBL PBL	18 9	12	28 10	25 18	23 2	27 11
081	Amherst Co Public Schools Ms Barbara Schnurer, Instructor *Chair's #: (804) 946-9386*	PO Box 410 Amherst	24521	2	HSE		SEC SEC	PBL PBL			Publication withheld			
037	Bedford County Schs-Mem Hosp Mrs Carolyn Roaf, Dir *Chair's #: (540) 587-5493*	1613 Oakwood St Bedford	24523		HSE		SEC SEC	PBL PBL	18	12	19 5	14 1	9 0	7 5
040	Buchanan County Sch Mrs Sandra Cook, Director *Chair's #: (540) 935-4541*	Rt 5 Box 110 Grundy	24614				SEC	PBL			Publication withheld			
015	Carilion Roanoke Mem Hosp Sch Mrs Carolyn W Lyon, Director *Chair's #: (540) 981-7362*	PO Box 13367 Roanoke	24033				HSP	PVT	12		17	26	12	21
074	Centra Hlth School of PN Mrs Patricia Uzsoy, Dean *Chair's #: (804) 947-3070*	1901 Tate Springs Rd Lynchburg	24503			A	IND	PVT	16	12	29	16	13	15
052	Central Sch-Norfolk Tech-Voc Center Miss Gloria Rudibaugh, Prog Leader *Chair's #: (757) 441-5625*	1330 N Military Hwy Norfolk	23502		HSE	A A	SEC SEC	PBL PBL	18	12	16 32	10 33	8 8	8 24
012	Charlottesvl-Albemrl-Tech Educ Center Mrs Joseph Jonhson, Dir *Chair's #: (804) 973-4461*	1000 E Rio Road Charlottesvil	22901				TCH	PVT	0		24	11	17	18

Explanation of footnotes on page x

VIRGINIA

- Continued

School Code	Name of School, Director of Program, and Phone Number	Street Address / City or Town and Zip Code	Footnotes	Type of Program	NLNAC Accreditation as of January 31, 1999	Administrative Control	Financial Support (principal source)	Number of Months in Program	Educational Requirements for Entering Adult Program	Enrollments as of October 15, 1998	Admissions Aug. 1, 1997 - July 31, 1998	Graduations Aug. 1, 1997 - July 31, 1998	Fall Admissions Aug. 1, 1998 - Dec. 31, 1998
048	Chesapeake Center for Science and Tech Mrs Kathleen A Jones, Director Chair's #: (757) 547-0134	1617 Cedar Rd Chesapeake 23322				SEC	PBL			18	15	12	6
067	Chesterfield Co Pub Schs Mrs Sandra Foote, Coord Chair's #: (804) 768-6160	10101 Courthouse Rd Chesterfield 23832				SEC	PBL			47	22	24	34
078	Computer Dynamics Inst, Inc Ms Kathleen Shovelin, Prog Manager Chair's #: (757) 499-4900 Ext 31	5361 Virginia Beach Blvd Virginia Beach 23462				TCH	PVT			155	117	80	79
038	Dabney S Lancaster Comm Coll Mrs Lisa Allison-Jones. Head Chair's #: (540)) 863-2843	PO Box 1000 Clifton Forge 24422	2,7			CC	PBL			Publication withheld			
011	Danville Comm College Mrs Lajuana Jordan, Director Chair's #: (804) 791-5356	1008 S Main St Danville 24541				CC	PBL	12	12	31	23	14	33
024	Fairfax Co School of PN Mrs Patricia Nelsen, Coord Chair's #: (703) 207-4011 Ext 4092	7423 Camp Alger Ave Falls Church 22042				SEC	PBL			Publication withheld			
013	Fredericksburg Area Sch of PN Mrs Sandra Demotses, Director Chair's #: (504) 891-0675	6713 Smith Station Rd Spotsylvania 22553		HSE		SEC SEC	PBL PBL	20	12	45 0	16 14	12 0	16 14
021	G Washington Carver-Piedmont Educ Ct Mrs Esther Frazier-Petty, Dir Chair's #: (540) 825-0476 Ext 08	PO Box 999 Culpeper 22701				TCH	PBL			Publication withheld			
050	Giles County Tech Center Mrs Nancy B Dowdy, Director Chair's #: (540) 921-1166 Ext 0016	PO Box 479 Pearisburg 24134		HSE		SEC SEC	PBL PBL	18 18	12 12	6 15	0 14	0 6	0 15
042	Henrico Co Schools-St Mary's Hospital Ms Ann L Unholz, Director Chair's #: (804) 328-4095	201 E Nine Mile Rd Highland Springs 23075		HS	A A	SEC SEC	PBL PBL		12	0 89	0 62	0 32	0 57
035	Henry Co Schs-Memorial Hosp Mrs Rebecca Greer, Dir Chair's #: (540) 656-0271	PO Box 5311 Martinsville 24115		HSE		SEC SEC	PBL PBL	18	12	32 4	26 8	27 7	25 8
062	Lafayette Sch of PN Mrs Karen Spangler, Coord Chair's #: (757) 565-4270	4460 Longhill Rd Williamsburg 23188		HSE		SEC SEC	PBL PBL	9 9	12	14 14	14 4	11 2	14 4
053	Lee County Voc Tech Sch Mrs Julia C Wyrick, Director Chair's #: (540) 346-1960	One Vo Tech Dr Box 100 Ben Hur 24218				SEC	PBL			57	28	27	39

VIRGINIA

- Continued

School Code	Name of School, Director of Program, and Phone Number	Street Address — City or Town and Zip Code		Footnotes	Type of Program	NLNAC Accreditation as of January 31, 1999	Administrative Control	Financial Support (principal source)	Number of Months in Program	Educational Requirements for Entering Adult Program	Enrollments as of October 15, 1998	Admissions Aug. 1, 1997 - July 31, 1998	Graduations Aug. 1, 1997 - July 31, 1998	Fall Admissions Aug. 1, 1998 - Dec. 31, 1998
005	Lord Fairfax Comm Coll Ms Betty Ward, Dir *Chair's #: (540) 722-3458*	156 Dowell J Circle Winchester	22602				CC	PBL	12		42	48	22	49
064	Loudoun Co Pub Schs-C Monroe V-T C Mrs Karen E Mason, Director *Chair's #: (703) 771-6560*	715 Childrens Ctr Rd SW Leesburg	20175		 HSE		TCH TCH	PBL PBL	18 18	12 12	32 10	19 6	12 5	14 5
059	Massanutten Tech Center Ms Linda Wood, Supv *Chair's #: (540) 434-5961 Ext 128*	325 Pleasant Valley Rd Harrisonburg	22801		 HSE		TCH TCH	PBL PBL	 18	 12	40 6	32 5	17 2	31 7
070	Medical Careers Inst Mrs Rose Saunders, Dir *Chair's #: (757) 497-8400*	5555 Greenwich Rd Suite106 Virginia Beach	23462				TCH	PVT	12	12	163	275	85	110
009	MedTech Hlth Care Training Ching Feng, Dir *Chair's #: (703) 360-3848*	8794 Sacramento Dr Alexandria	22309	2			TCH	PBL			Publication withheld			
010	New Horizon Reg Educ Center Mrs Suzanne Bolt, Coord *Chair's #: (757) 766-1100 Ext 336*	520 Butler Farm Rd Hampton	23666		 HSE	A A	TCH TCH	PBL PBL	18 18	12 12	0 61	0 57	0 57	0 67
025	New River Comm College Mrs LaRue Ridenhour, Prog Head *Chair's #: (540) 674-3600 Ext 251*	PO Box 1127 Dublin	24084				CC	PBL	12	12	28	30	15	29
029	Page County Tech Center Mrs Jessica Ressler, Dir *Chair's #: (540) 778-4276*	525 Middleburg Rd Luray	22835	2	 HSE		SEC SEC	PBL PBL	 18	 12	6 4	0 0	8 0	6 4
016	Petersburg City Schs-Southside Reg Mrs Jean Riddle, Coord *Chair's #: (804) 862-7022*	816 E Bank St Petersburg	23803		 HSE		SEC SEC	PBL PBL		 11	31 7	36 2	8 0	39 9
044	Portsmouth Public Sch of PN Mrs Katherine B Decker, Director *Chair's #: (757) 393-5408*	3701 Willett Dr Portsmouth	23707				TCH	PBL			Publication withheld			
001	Prince William Co Schs Ms Bette Sneed, Dir *Chair's #: (703) 791-7357*	PO Box 389 Manassas	20108		 HSE		SEC SEC	PBL PBL	 18		0 75	0 50	0 27	0 0
058	Radford City PN Sch Mrs Virginia Graham Jones, Dir *Chair's #: (540) 731-3669*	PO Box 3698 Radford	24143		 HSE		SEC SEC	PBL PBL			Publication withheld			
071	Rappahannock Comm College Mrs Dianne Lucy, Prog Head *Chair's #: (804) 758-6779*	12745 College Dr Glenns	23149				CC	PBL	12	12	26	34	30	27

Explanation of footnotes on page x

School Code	Name of School, Director of Program, and Phone Number	Street Address / City or Town and Zip Code	Footnotes	Type of Program	NLNAC Accreditation as of January 31, 1999	Administrative Control	Financial Support (principal source)	Number of Months in Program	Educational Requirements for Entering Adult Program	Enrollments as of October 15, 1998	Admissions Aug. 1, 1997 - July 31, 1998	Graduations Aug. 1, 1997 - July 31, 1998	Fall Admissions Aug. 1, 1998 - Dec. 31, 1998
	VIRGINIA												
	- Continued												
043	Richmond Public Schools / Mrs Hilda Roundtree, Instr Spec / Chair's #: (804) 780-6076	2020 Westwood Ave / Richmond 23230			A	TCH	PBL			Publication withheld			
				HS	A	TCH	PBL						
				HSE	A	TCH	PBL		12				
051	Richmond Sch of Hlth and Tech / Ms M Fretheim. Dir / Chair's #: (804) 780-0167	421 E Franklin St Box 2111 / Richmond 23218	2			TCH	PVT			Publication withheld			
027	Riverside Hlth System & Newpt News S / Mrs Brenda Booth, Coord / Chair's #: (757) 594-2720	12420 Warwick Blvd / Newport News 23606			A	SEC	PBL	11	12	28	33	25	29
				HSE	A	SEC	PBL	20	12	6	16	0	6
004	Russell Co Voc Sch of PN / Mrs Kimberley Israel, Dir / Chair's #: (540) 889-6547	1 Vocational Sch Rd Box 849 / Lebanon 24266				TCH	PBL			30	30	12	0
				HSE		TCH	PBL	18	12	6	6	0	0
079	Salem Sch of PN / Mrs Martha Barnas, Prog Head / Chair's #: (540) 847-6283	400 N Spartan Dr / Salem 24153				CC	PBL			Publication withheld			
030	Scott Co Voc Center / Mrs Brigitte Casteel, Dir / Chair's #: (540) 386-6515	150 Broadwater / Gate City 24251				TCH	PBL	18		37	26	18	25
				HSE		TCH	PBL	18		5	4	1	5
014	Shore Memoral Hospital / Mrs Bonnie R Nordstrom, Director / Chair's #: (757) 442-8771	PO Box 17 10098 Rogers Dr / Nassawadox 23413				HSP	PVT	12	12	16	13	12	15
041	Smyth County Voc Sch of PN / Ms Georgia Miller, Dir / Chair's #: (540) 646-8117	Rt 2 Box 653 / Marion 24354				TCH	PBL			0	0	0	0
033	Southampton Mem Hosp / Mrs Ercelle Vann, Dir / Chair's #: (757) 569-6414	100 Fairview Dr / Franklin 23851				HSP	PBL	12	12	14	15	15	14
046	Southside Sch of PN / Mrs Pamela Fowler, Dir / Chair's #: (804) 315-2630	800 Oak Street / Farmville 23901	2			TCH	PBL	12	12	20	20	19	20
073	Southside VA Comm College / Ms Shirley Bugg, Prof / Chair's #: (804) 949-1037	109 Campus Dr / Alberta 23821				CC	PBL			Publication withheld			
002	Southside VA Comm College / Mrs Annie Lee Owen, Dir / Chair's #: (804) 575-3100 Ext 320	2204 Wilborn Ave / South Boston 24592				CC	PBL			27	27	17	27
034	Stonewall Jackson Hosp / Mrs Penny Fauber-Moore, Director / Chair's #: (540) 462-1351	One Health Circle / Lexington 24450				TCH	PBL	11	12	15	16	9	0

Explanation of footnotes on page x

School Code	Name of School, Director of Program, and Phone Number	Street Address City or Town and Zip Code	Footnotes	Type of Program	NLNAC Accreditation as of January 31, 1999	Administrative Control	Financial Support (principal source)	Number of Months in Program	Educational Requirements for Entering Adult Program	Enrollments as of October 15, 1998	Admissions Aug. 1, 1997 - July 31, 1998	Graduations Aug. 1, 1997 - July 31, 1998	Fall Admissions Aug. 1, 1998 - Dec. 31, 1998
	VIRGINIA												
	- Continued												
020	Suffolk Public Sch-Obici Mem Hosp Ms Gwen T Sweat, Director Chair's #: (757) 934-4826	L Obici Mem Hosp Box 1100 Suffolk 23439			A	HSP	PBL	12	12	11	21	17	0
003	Tazewell Co Career Tech Center Ms Dolores Mulkey, Director Chair's #: (540) 596-6650	2949 W Front St Richlands 24641		HSE		TCH TCH	PBL PBL	18	12	0 18	0 38	0 17	0 41
068	Twin Co Sch of PN/WCC Mr Jeffrey Miller, Prog Head Chair's #: (540) 238-1177	121 W Grayson St Galax 24333				CC	PBL			Publication withheld			
006	Valley Voc-Tech Ctr Sch of Nsg Mrs G G Hildebrand, Director Chair's #: (540) 245-5002	Rt 3 Box 265 Fisherville 22939				TCH	PBL			25	33	10	24
060	Virginia Beach Sch of PN Ms Rose Mary Saliba, Director Chair's #: (757) 427-5300	2925 N Landing Rd Virginia Beach 23456		HSE	A A	TCH TCH	PBL PBL	24 18	12 12	50 29	21 39	16 14	17 28
049	Virginia Western Comm Coll Mrs Martha Barnas, Prog Head Chair's #: (540) 857-6283	Po Box 14007 Roanoke 24038	2	HS HSE		CC CC CC	PBL PBL PBL	18 18	12 12	25 1	17 5	0 0	17 1
054	Washington County Schs Mrs Margaret B Humphreys, Dir Chair's #: (540) 628-1870	255 Stanley St Abingdon 24210		HSE		TCH TCH	PBL PBL	18	12 12	28 6	20 6	13 0	21 6
018	Wise County Voc Tech Sch of PN Ms Jennifer Hall, Dir Chair's #: (540) 328-6113	PO Box 1218 Wise 24293				SEC	PBL			Publication withheld			
	WASHINGTON												
	25 Programs in 23 Schools												
003	Bates Technical College Mr Jeffrey Bonnell, Dir Chair's #: (253) 596-1617	1101 S Yakima Ave Tacoma 98405				TCH	PBL			80	109	50	54
015	Bellingham Tech Coll Ms Ruby Mans, Coord Chair's #: (360) 738-3105 Ext 432	3028 Lindbergh Ave Bellingham 98225				TCH	PBL	15	12	97	80	30	24
026	Big Bend Comm College Mrs Linda Wrynn, Dir Chair's #: (509) 762-6285	Moses Lake 98837				CC	PBL	11	12	21	14	11	14
011	Centralia College Ms Nola Ormond, Dir Chair's #: (360) 736-9391 Ext 449	600 West Locust Centralia 98531				CC	PBL	11	12	27	26	27	27

Explanation of footnotes on page x

School Code	Name of School, Director of Program, and Phone Number	Street Address City or Town and Zip Code	Footnotes	Type of Program	NLNAC Accreditation as of January 31, 1999	Administrative Control	Financial Support (principal source)	Number of Months in Program	Educational Requirements for Entering Adult Program	Enrollments as of October 15, 1998	Admissions Aug. 1, 1997 - July 31, 1998	Graduations Aug. 1, 1997 - July 31, 1998	Fall Admissions Aug. 1, 1998 - Dec. 31, 1998
	WASHINGTON												
	- Continued												
007	Clark College Mrs Dot Nicholes, Interim Director *Chair's #: (360) 992-2192*	1800 E McLoughlin Blvd Vancouver 98663				CC	PBL	12	12	20	20	13	20
021	Clover Park Tech Coll Mrs Sheila Reilly, Dir *Chair's #: (253) 589-5536*	4500 Steilacoom Blvd, SW Lakewood Center 98499				TCH	PBL			119	125	66	58
013	Columbia Basin College Ms Donna E Campbell, Dean *Chair's #: (509) 547-0511 Ext 283*	2600 N 20th Pasco 99301	7			CC	PBL			Data reported w/AD prog			
005	Everett Community College Mr Stuart Barger, Director *Chair's #: (425) 388-9399*	801 Wetmore Ave Everett 98201	7			CC	PBL			Data reported w/AD prog			
010	Grays Harbor Coll Dr Candice Mohar, Chair *Chair's #: (360) 538-4148*	1620 Edwards Smith Dr Aberdeen 98520				CC	PBL	12	12	16	16	14	16
027	Green River Comm College Ms Julia Short, Coordinator *Chair's #: (206) 833-9111*	12401 SE 320th St Auburn 98002				CC	PBL			Publication withheld			
037	Lake Washington Tech College Ms Patricia Stuart, Coord *Chair's #: (425) 739-8371*	11605 132nd Ave NE Kirkland 98034				TCH	PBL			Data reported w/AD prog			
014	Lower Columbia College Ms Helen Hing, Director *Chair's #: (360) 577-3446*	1600 Maple Longview 98632	7			CC	PBL			Data reported w/AD Prog			
030	North Seattle Comm College Ms Sandra Liming, Coord *Chair's #: (206) 527-3791*	9600 College Way, N Seattle 98103				CC	PBL			Publication withheld			
034	Oak Harbor PN Prog-Skagit Valley Coll Ms Kathleen A Petet, Dept Chair *Chair's #: (360) 679-5324*	1900 SE Pioneer Way Oak Harbor 98277				CC	PBL			Publication withheld			
004	Olympic College Mrs Marge Herzog, Coord *Chair's #: (360) 475-7751*	1600 Chester Ave Bremerton 98310	7			CC	PBL			Data reported w/AD Prog			
036	Renton Technical College Ms Toni Whitefield, Assoc Dean *Chair's #: (425) 235-2352 Ext 5552*	3000 NE 4th St Renton 98056				TCH	PBL	11	12	54	64	25	36
012	Skagit Valley College Mrs Flora G Adams, Chair *Chair's #: (360) 416-7631*	2405 College Way Mount Vernon 98273	7			CC	PBL			Data reported w/AD prog			

Explanation of footnotes on page x

School Code	Name of School, Director of Program, and Phone Number	Street Address / City or Town and Zip Code		Footnotes	Type of Program	NLNAC Accreditation as of January 31, 1999	Administrative Control	Financial Support (principal source)	Number of Months in Program	Educational Requirements for Entering Adult Program	Enrollments as of October 15, 1998	Admissions Aug. 1, 1997 - July 31, 1998	Graduations Aug. 1, 1997 - July 31, 1998	Fall Admissions Aug. 1, 1998 - Dec. 31, 1998
	WASHINGTON													
	- Continued													
032	South Puget Sound Comm College Ms Ruby Flesner, Director *Chair's #: (360) 754-7711 Ext 285*	2011 Mottman Rd, SW Olympia	98502				CC	PBL	11	12	24	24	20	24
002	Spokane Comm Coll Mrs Carol Nelson, Dir *Chair's #: (509) 533-7311*	N 1810 Greene St Spokane	99207	7			CC	PBL			Data reported w/AD prog			
017	Walla Walla Comm College (2 Branches Mrs Marilyn Galusha, Dir *Chair's #: (509) 527-4240*	500 Tausick Way Walla Walla	99362	7			CC	PBL			Data reported w/AD prog			
008	Wenatchee Valley College Ms Connie Barnes, Dir *Chair's #: (509) 664-2532*	1300 5th St Wenatchee	98801	7			CC	PBL			Data reported w/AD prog			
035	Wenatchee Vly College-Omak Branch Mrs Connie Barnes, Director *Chair's #: (509) 665-2605*	1300 So 5th Wenatchee	98801	7			CC	PBL			Data reported w/AD prog			
006	Yakima Valley College Miss Rhoda Taylor, Dept Head *Chair's #: (509) 574-4909*	PO Box 22520 Yakima	98907	7			CC	PBL			Data reported w /AD prog			
	WEST VIRGINIA													
	20 Programs in 20 Schools													
006	Academy Career Technology Ms Ella Pennington, Coord *Chair's #: (304) 256-4615 Ext 4675*	390 Stanaford Rd Beckley	25801				TCH	PBL	12	12	39	35	30	40
001	B M Spurr Sch of Practical Nursing Mrs Carol Storm, Director *Chair's #: (304) 843-3255*	800 Wheeling Ave Glen Dale	26038			A	HSP	PVT	12	12	22	18	17	21
005	Cabell Co Voc-Tech Ctr Ms Sandra Thompson, Chair *Chair's #: (304) 528-5108*	1035 Norway Ave Huntington	25705				TCH	PBL			30	30	21	30
027	Fred W Eberle School of Practical Nsg Mrs Deborah Carpenter, Coord *Chair's #: (304) 472-1276*	Rt 5 Box 2 Buckhannon	26201				TCH	PBL	12	12	14	21	15	0
002	Garnet Career Ctr Sch of Practical Nsg Mrs Mary Brothers, Coord *Chair's #: (304) 348-6114*	422 Dickinson St Charleston	25301			A	TCH	PBL			Publication withheld			
010	James Rumsey Tech Inst Mrs Mary Ann Shackelford, Coord *Chair's #: (304) 754-7925 Ext 0036*	Rt 6, Box 268 Martinsburg	25401				TCH	PBL	12	12	25	31	21	0

Explanation of footnotes on page x

School Code	Name of School, Director of Program, and Phone Number	Street Address City or Town and Zip Code		Footnotes	Type of Program	NLNAC Accreditation as of January 31, 1999	Administrative Control	Financial Support (principal source)	Number of Months in Program	Educational Requirements for Entering Adult Program	Enrollments as of October 15, 1998	Admissions Aug. 1, 1997 - July 31, 1998	Graduations Aug. 1, 1997 - July 31, 1998	Fall Admissions Aug. 1, 1998 - Dec. 31, 1998
	WEST VIRGINIA													
	- Continued													
018	Logan-Mingo Sch of PN Mrs Marlene V Newsome, Coord *Chair's #: (304) 752-4687 Ext 4187*	Box 1747 Logan	25601				TCH	PBL			33	34	19	33
019	McDowell Co Voc-Tech Ctr Mrs Francine Kirby, Coord *Chair's #: (304) 436-6180*	Drawer V Welch	24801				TCH	PVT			23	23	23	28
008	Mercer County Voc-Tech Ctr Ms Sandra Thompson, Coord *Chair's #: (304) 425-9551*	1397 Staffinal Dr Princeton	24740				TCH	PBL			Publication withheld			
076	Mineral County Voc Sch of PN Ms Rita Jean Harber, Coord *Chair's #: (304) 788-4240 Ext 17*	600 South Water St Keyser	26726				TCH	PBL			Publication withheld			
029	Mingo Co Voc Sch of PN Ms Teresa Anne Carter, Dir *Chair's #: (304) 475-2078*	Rt 2 Box 52-A Delbarton	25670				TCH	PBL			22	30	22	0
007	Monongalia Co Voc-Tech Ctr Mrs Lynda Overking, Coord *Chair's #: (304) 291-9240 Ext 22*	1000 Mississippi St Morgantown	26505				TCH	PBL	12	12	22	30	20	30
031	Randoph County Voc Tech Center Mrs Robin Riggleman, Coord *Chair's #: (304) 636-9195*	200 Kennedy Drive Elkins	26441				TCH	PBL	12	12	16	25	20	0
023	Region IV Sch of PN Mrs. Rebbecca Edwards, Coord *Chair's #: (304) 647-6487*	One Spartan Lane Lewisburg	24901				TCH	PBL	12	12	21	16	14	22
022	Roane-Jackson Tech Center Ms Donita Young, Coord *Chair's #: (304) 372-7335*	4800 Spencer Rd Leroy	25252				TCH	PBL	12	12	24	26	18	0
020	Summers County Voc Sch Mrs Judith Long, Coord *Chair's #: (304) 466-6040 Ext 128*	116 Main St Hinton	25951				TCH	PBL	12	12	22	22	13	22
013	United Tech Center Sch of PN Mrs Monica Iaquinta, Facilitator *Chair's #: (304) 624-3284*	Rt 3, Box 43C Clarksburg	26301				TCH	PBL			Publication withheld			
017	Wood County Vocational School Mrs Carolyn Edwards, Coord *Chair's #: (304) 420-9651 Ext 264*	1515 Blizzard Dr Parkersburg	26101			A	TCH	PBL	12	12	23	30	27	30
024	Wyoming Co Voc Sch Ms Susan Browning, Coord *Chair's #: (304) 732-8050 Ext 105*	HCr 72 Box 200 HCR Pineville	24874				TCH	PBL			28	27	20	0

Explanation of footnotes on page x

School Code	Name of School, Director of Program, and Phone Number	Street Address City or Town and Zip Code	Footnotes	Type of Program	NLNAC Accreditation as of January 31, 1999	Administrative Control	Financial Support (principal source)	Number of Months in Program	Educational Requirements for Entering Adult Program	Enrollments as of October 15, 1998	Admissions Aug. 1, 1997 - July 31, 1998	Graduations Aug. 1, 1997 - July 31, 1998	Fall Admissions Aug. 1, 1998 - Dec. 31, 1998
	WISCONSIN												
	12 Programs in 12 Schools												
017	Blackhawk Tech College Ms Beth Oren, Assoc Dean *Chair's #: (608) 757-7678*	6004 Prairie Rd PO Box 5009 Janesville 53547	7			TCH	PBL			Data reported w/AD prog			
013	Chippewa Valley Tech College Ms M Dickens-Grosskopf , Dir *Chair's #: (715) 833-6419*	620 W Clairemont Ave Eau Claire 54701				TCH	PBL			Publication withheld			
003	Fox Valley Tech College Mrs Ardythe Korpela, Dept Chair *Chair's #: (920) 735-5664*	1825 N Bluemound Dr Appleton 54913				TCH	PBL	11	10	37	55	25	47
015	Gateway Tech Coll Mrs Kathleen Russ, Dean *Chair's #: (414) 656-6934*	3520 30th Ave Kenosha 53144				TCH	PBL	9	12	50	40	39	20
012	Lakeshore Tech College Ms Nancy Kaprelian, Dean *Chair's #: (920) 458-4183 Ext 0180*	1290 North Ave Cleveland 53015	7			TCH	PBL			Data reported w/AD prog			
004	Madison Area Tech College Ms Alda Preston, Assoc Dean *Chair's #: (608) 246-6014*	3550 Anderson St Madison 53704			A	TCH	PBL			Publication withheld			
002	Milwaukee Area Tech College Dr Nancy Vrabec, Assoc Dean *Chair's #: (414) 297-6241*	700 W State St Milwaukee 53233			A	TCH	PBL	12	12	185	110	68	55
007	Moraine Park Tech College Ms Linda Walter, Assoc Dean *Chair's #: (414) 335-5720*	700 Gould St Beaver Dam 53916			A	CC	PBL	10	12	51	59	39	37
008	NE Wisconsin Tech College Ms Carol Rafferty, Assoc Dean *Chair's #: (920) 498-5482 Ext 5482*	2740 W Mason St Box 19042 Green Bay 54307				TCH	PBL	11	12	46	23	23	46
014	SW Wisconsin Tech College Ms Sharon Selleck-Lehman, Dean *Chair's #: (608) 822-3262 Ext 2151*	1800 Bronson Blvd Fennimore 53809	7			TCH	PBL	10	12	20	23	16	20
011	Waukesha County Tech College Dr Kitty Gotham, Assoc Dean *Chair's #: (414) 691-5368*	800 Main St Pewaukee 53072	6			TCH	PBL			Publication withheld			
016	Western Wisconsin Tech Coll Ms Donna Haggard, Chair *Chair's #: (608) 785-9186*	304 N 6th St La Crosse 54602	6			TCH	PBL			Publication withheld			

Explanation of footnotes on page x

School Code	Name of School, Director of Program, and Phone Number	Street Address City or Town and Zip Code		Footnotes	Type of Program	NLNAC Accreditation as of January 31, 1999	Administrative Control	Financial Support (principal source)	Number of Months in Program	Educational Requirements for Entering Adult Program	Enrollments as of October 15, 1998	Admissions Aug. 1, 1997 - July 31, 1998	Graduations Aug. 1, 1997 - July 31, 1998	Fall Admissions Aug. 1, 1998 - Dec. 31, 1998
	WYOMING													
	6 Programs in 6 Schools													
001	Casper College Mrs Judith Turner, Dir *Chair's #: (307) 268-2233*	125 College Dr Casper	82601	7			CC	PBL			Data reported w/AD prog			
003	Laramie County Comm College Ms Jan Freudenthal, Coord *Chair's #: (307) 778-1133*	1400 E College Dr Cheyenne	82007	7		A	CC	PBL			Data reported w\AD prog			
007	Northern Wyoming Comm College PN P Mrs Nancy Larmer, Director *Chair's #: (307) 686-0254 Ext 227*	750 W 8th Suite 1 Gillette	82716				CC	PBL	9	12	19	23	0	0
005	Northwest College Mr William Clinton, Dir *Chair's #: (307) 754-6479*	231 W 6th Powell	82435	7		A	CC	PBL			Data reported w/ AD prog			
004	Sheridan College Mrs Trudy Munsick Acting Dir *Chair's #: (307) 674-6446 Ext 6153*	PO Box 1500 Sheridan	82801				CC	PBL			Data reported w/AD prog			
006	Western Wyoming Comm College Ms Karen Medina, Dir *Chair's #: (307) 382-1801*	PO Box 428 Rock Springs	82901	7			CC	PBL			Data reported with /AD pro			

SUMMARY TABLES

New LPN/LVN Schools

(between October 16, 1997and October 15, 1998)

STATE	NAME OF SCHOOL	CITY or TOWN	TYPE OF PROGRAM
CA	Nursing Care Providers Vocational School Pacific College Tri - County ROP San Joaquin Valley College Visalia Adult School	San Bruno Costa Mesa Yuba City Visalia Visalia	Adult Adult Adult Adult Adult
KS	North Central Kansas Area Technical College	Hays	Adult
MD	Baltimore City Community Center Chesapeake College	Baltimore Wye Mills	Adult Adult
MO	Case Career Center	Harrinsonville	Adult
OH	Central Ohio Technical School Lima Technical College	Newark Lima	Adult Adult
PR	Ponce Technical School Ramirez College of Business and Technology Rosslyn Training Academy	Ponce Hato Rey Aguada	Adult Adult Adult
TX	Angelina College Childress Regional Medical Center El Paso Community College Institute for Health Career Development South Texas Community College Vangard Institute of Technology	Jasper Childress El Paso Fort Worth Weslasco Edinburg	Adult Adult Adult Adult Adult Adult
VA	Amherst Community Public School Richmond School of Health and Technology	Amherst Richmond	HE Adult
UT	Davis Applied Technology Center	Kaysville	Adult

Closed LPN/LVN Schools

(between October 16, 1997 and October 15, 1998)

STATE	NAME OF SCHOOL	CITY or TOWN	TYPE OF PROGRAM	NLNAC ACCREDITATION STATUS	ADMINISTRATION CONTROL	FINANCIAL SUPPORT	GRADUATIONS:AUG.1,1997- JULY31, 1998
GA	Putnam County Public School	Eatonton	Adult	-	HSP	PBL	-
IL	Jacksonville School of PN Board of Education District 117	Jacksonville	Adult	-	SEC	PVT	-
NJ	Bergen Pines County Hospital	Paramus	Adult	A	SEC	PBL	-
NY	Iona College	New Rochelle	Adult	A	COL	PVT	-
PA	Chester Upland School District Warren County Area Vocational Technical School	Chester Warren	Adult Adult	- A	SEC Tech	PBL PBL	- -
TX	Jasper Memorial Hospital Kilgore College Paris Junior College San Jacinto College UTB/TSC-TX Southmont College	Jasper Kilgore Paris Houston Weslasco	Adult Adult Adult Adult Adult	- - - - -	SEC CC COL COL COL	PBL PBL PBL PBL PBL	- - - - -
VA	Commonwealth Technical Institute Greensville County Memorial Hospital	Virginia Beach Emporia	Adult Adult	- -	Tech HSP	PVT PBL	- -
WVA	West Virginia Northern Community College	Wheeling	Adult	-	COL	PBL	-

DIRECTORY OF
BOARDS OF NURSING

DIRECTORY OF
BOARDS OF NURSING

Judi Crume, Exec. Off.
Alabama Board of Nursing
Montgomery, Alabama 36130-3900
Tel (334) 242-4296

Dorothy Fulton, Exec. Admin.
Alaska Board of Nursing
3601 "C" St., Suite 722
Anchorage, Alaska 99503
Tel (907) 269-8161

Mrs. Repekam Howland, Exec. Sec
Health Services Regulatory Board
LBJ Tropical Medical Center
Pago Pago, American Samoa 96799
Tel (684) 633-1222

Joey Ridenour, Exec. Dir.
Arizona State Board of Nursing
1651 E. Morton, Suite 150
Phoenix, Arizona 85020
Tel (602) 331-8111 ext. 139

Faith Fields, Exec. Dir.
Arkansas State Board of Nursing
1123 South Univ., Suite 800
Little Rock, Arkansas 72204
Tel (501) 686-2700

Teresa Bello Jones, Exec. Off.
Board of VN & Psych. Tech. Examiners
2535 Capitol Oaks Dr., Suite 205
Sacramento, California 95833-2919
Tel (916) 263-7840

Janet Zubreni, Acting Prog Admin.
Colorado State Board of Nursing
1560 Broadway, Suite 670
Denver, Colorado 80202-2410
Tel (303) 894-2819

Wendy Furniss, Supr.
Department of Public Health
Board of Examiners for Nursing
410 Capital Ave.
P.O. Box 340308
Hartford, Connecticut 06134-0308
Tel (860) 509-7400

Iva J. Boardman, Exec. Dir.
Delaware Board of Nursing
Cannon Bldg., P.O. Box 1401
Dover, Delaware 19901
Tel (302) 739-4522, Ext. 217

Barbara .W. Hagans, Contact Rep
District of Columbia Board of Nursing
825 North Capital NE Rm. 2224
Washington D. C. 20002
Tel (202) 442-9200

Dr Ruth Stiehl, Exec Dir.
Florida State Board of Nursing
4080 Woodcock Dr., Suite 202
Jacksonville, Florida 32207
Tel (904) 858-6961

Janet M. Starr, Nsg. Educ. Consultant
Georgia Board of Examiner of
 Licensed Practical Nurse
166 Pryor St., NW, Suite 300
Atlanta, Georgia 30303
Tel (404) 656-3921

Teo-Fila Cruz, Exec. Dir.
Guam Board of Nurse Examiners
P.O. Box 2816
Agana, Guam 96910
Tel (671) 734-7295

Kathleen Yokouchi, Exec Off.
Hawaii Board of Nursing
Box 3469
Honolulu, Hawaii 99503
Tel (671) 734-7295

Sandra Evans, Asst. Exec. Dir.
Idaho State Board of Nursing
P.O. Box 83720
Boise, Idaho 83720-0061
Tel (208) 334-3110 Ext. 34

Elizabeth Cleinmark, Acting Coord.
Department of Professional Regulation
320 W. Washington St.
Springfield, Illinois 62786
Tel (317) 785-9465

Gina Voorhies, Dir.
Indiana State Board of Nursing
402 West Washington Street
Indianapolis, Indiana 46204
Tel (317) 233-4405

Lorinda Inman, Exec, Dir.
Iowa Board of Nursing
1223 E. Court Avenue
Des Moines, Iowa 50319
Tel (515) 281-4828

Pat Johnson, Exec. Admin.
Kansas State Board of Nursing
900 SW Jackson St., Suite 551S
Topeka, Kansas 66612-1256
Tel (785) 296-3782

Sharon M. Weisenbeck, Exec. Dir.
Kentucky Board of Nursing
312 Whittington Pky., Suite 300
Louisville, Kentucky 40222-5172
Tel (502) 329-7033

Terry L. Demarcay, Exec. Dir.
Louisiana State Board of
 Practical Nurse Examiners
3421 N Causeway Blvd., Suite 203
Metarie, Louisiana 70002-5791
Tel (504) 838-5791

Myra Broadway, Exec. Dir.
Maine State Board of Nursing
24 Stone St House Station 158
Augusta, Maine 04333-0158
Tel (207) 287-1133

Donna Dorsey, Exec. Dir.
Maryland Board of Nursing
4140 Patterson Ave.
Baltimore, Maryland 21215-2254
Tel (410) 585-1924

Theresa M. Bonanno, Exec. Dir.
Board of Registration in Nursing
100 Cambridge St., Room 150
Boston, Massachusetts 02202
Tel (617) 727-3060

Mary A Vanden Bosch, Nurse Consultant
Michigan Board of Nursing
P.O. Box 30018, 611 West Ottawa
Lansing, Michigan 48909
Tel (517) 373-4674

Joyce M. Schowalter, Exec. Dir.
Minnesota Board of Nursing
2829 University Ave., SE # 500
Minneapolis, Minnesota 55114-3253
Tel (612) 617-2294

Sandra Bates, Coord
Health Science Technology
Office of Vocational-Tech Education
Department of Education, P.O. Box 771
Jackson, Mississippi 39205-0771
Tel (601) 359-3461

Marcia Flesner, Exec. Dir
Missouri State Board of Nursing
3605 Missouri Blvd., Box 656
Jefferson City, Missouri 65102-0656
Tel (573) 751-0080

Dianne Wickham, Exec. Dir.
Montana State Board of Nursing
111 Jackson, Arcade Bldg.
Helena, Montana 59620-0513
Tel (406) 444-2071

Charlene Kelley, Assoc. Dir.
Bureau of Examining Board
P.O. Box 95007
Lincoln, Nebraska 68509
Tel (402) 471-4917

Kathy Apple, Exec. Dir.
Nevada State Board of Nursing
4335 S. Industrial Rd. # 420
Las Vegas, Nevada 89103
Tel (702) 688-2620

Doris G. Nuttelman, Exec. Dir.
State Board of Nursing
78 Regional Dr. P.O. Box 3898
Concord, Hew Hampshire 03301
Tel (603) 271-2323

Patricia Polansky, Exec. Dir.
New Jersey Board of Nursing
P.O. Box 45010
Newark, New Jersey 07101
Tel (973) 504-6499

Dr. Debra Brady, Exec Dir.
New Mexico Board of Nursing
4206 Louisiana NE, Suite A
Albuquerque, New Mexico 87109
Tel (505) 841-8340

Milene A Sower, Exec. Sec.
New York State Board for Nursing
The Cultural Center, Room 3023
Albany, New York 12230
Tel (518) 486-2967

Mary P. Johnson, Exec. Dir.
North Carolina Board of Nursing
P.O. Box 2129
Raleigh, North Carolina 27602
Tel (919) 782-3211

Dr Constance Kalanek, Exec. Dir.
North Dakota Board of Nursing
919 S. 7th St., Suite 504
Bismarck, North Dakota 58504-5881
Tel (701) 328-9781

Dorothy Fiorino, Exec. Dir.
Ohio Board of Nursing
77 S. High St.17th Floor
Columbus, Ohio 43266-0316
Tel (614) 466-9800

Sulinda Moffett, Exec. Dir.
Oklahoma Board of Nursing
2915 N. Classen Blvd., Suite 524
Oklahoma City, Oklahoma 73106
Tel (405) 962-1800

Joan Bouchard, Exec. Dir.
Oregon State Board of Nursing
800 N.E. Oregon St., #25
Portland, Oregon 97232
Tel (503) 731-4745

Miriam H. Limo, Exec. Sec.
Pennsylvania State Board of Nurses
P.O. Box 2649
Harrisburg, Pennsylvania 17105
Tel (717) 783-7142

Angel Canales, Dir.
General Council on Education
P.O. Box 195429
San Juan, Puerto Rico 00919-5429
Tel (787) 764-0101 Ext. 236

Nikki Deary, Interim Dir.
Board of Nursing Education &
 Nurse Registration
3 Capitol Hill, Rm. 105
Providence, Rhode Island 02908-5097
Tel (401) 277-2827

Adrienne Youmans, Acting Admin.
State Board of Nursing for South Carolina
P.O. Box 12367
Columbia, South Carolina 29211-2367
Tel (803) 896-4532

Dianna Vander-Woude, Exec Sec.
South Dakota Board of Nursing
4300 South Louis Ave Suite C1
Sioux Falls, South Dakota 57106
Tel (605) 362-2760

Elizabeth J. Lund, Exec. Dir.
Tennessee Board of Nursing
425 Fifth Ave. N.
Nashville Tennessee 37247-1010
Tel (615) 741-1445

Mary Strange, Exec. Dir.
Board of Vocational Nurse Examiners
333 Guadeloupe St., Suite 3-100
Tel (512) 305-8100, Ext.205

Laura Poe, Exec. Admin.
Utah State Board of Nursing
160 E. 300 South Box 146741
Salt Lake City, Utah 84114-6741
Tel (801) 530-6789

Anita Ristau, Exec. Dir.
Vermont Board of Nursing
Licensing and Registration Div.
109 State St.
Montpelier, Vermont 05602
Tel (802) 828-2396

Winifred Garfield, Exec Dir.
Virgin Island Boards of Nurse Licensure
P.O. Box 4247
Charlotte Amalie, Virgin Islands 00803
Tel (340) 776-7397

Nancy K. Durrett, Exec. Dir.
Virginia Board of Nursing
6606 W. Broad St., 4Th Floor
Richmond, Virginia 23230-117
Tel (804) 662-9951

Paula Meyer, Exec Dir.
Washington State Nursing Care
Quality Assurance Commission
1300 Quince, P.O. Box 47864
Olympia, Washington 98504-7864
Tel (360) 236-4713

Nancy R. Wilson, Exec. Sec.
West Virginia State Board of
Examiners for Licensed Practical Nurses
101 Dee Drive.
Charleston, West Virginia 25311-1688
Tel (304) 348-3572

Thomas A. Neumann, Educ. Off.
Wisconsin Department of
Regulation & Licensing
P.O. Box 8935
Madison, Wisconsin 53708-8935
Tel (608) 267-2357

Mary Sharper, Interim Exec. Dir.
State of Wyoming Board of Nursing
2020 Carey Ave Suite 110
Cheyenne, Wyoming 82002
Tel (307) 777-6127

Get on the fast-track to nursing school with this invaluable test-prep tool!

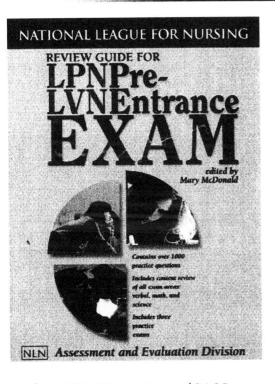

NATIONAL LEAGUE FOR NURSING

REVIEW GUIDE FOR
LPN Pre-LVN Entrance EXAM

edited by
Mary McDonald

Contains over 1000 practice questions

Includes content review of all exam areas: verbal, math, and science

Includes three practice exams

NLN Assessment and Evaluation Division

October 1999, 200 pp., Paper, $24.95,
ISBN 0-7637-1061-X
Prices are subject to change without notice.

This comprehensive review guide will help you to prepare for a nursing school entrance exam. The books' design, content review, and test questions, have been carefully organized to help you prepare for this this important test. A bibliography is included for those who seek further review of specific topics. In addition, the introduction explains the educational opportunities that are available in nursing and provides a helpful study guide and test-taking tips.

Features:

- Contains over 1,000 practice questions
- Extensive review is provided for each of the subjects tested on the exams — verbal, math, and science
- Contains valuable information on study skills, scholarships, and much more
- Includes three practice exams

Mail, phone, fax, or e-mail your order to:

Jones and Bartlett Publishers
Attn: Marketing Department
40 Tall Pine Drive
Sudbury, MA 01776
800-832-0034
Fax: 978-443-8000
E-mail: info@jbpub.com
www.jbpub.com

EXPERIENCE THE DIFFERENCE
www.jbpub.com

src:lpn/lvn99